BED
NUMBER
TEN

BED NUMBER TEN

Sue Baier and Mary Zimmeth

HOLT, RINEHART AND WINSTON   NEW YORK

First published in February 1986 by Holt, Rinehart and
Winston, 383 Madison Avenue, New York, New York 10017.
Published simultaneously in Canada by Holt, Rinehart
and Winston of Canada, Limited.

Library of Congress Cataloging-in-Publication Data
Baier, Sue.
Bed number ten.
1. Baier, Sue—Health.   2. Polyradiculoneuritis—Pa-
tients—United States—Biography.   I. Zimmeth, Mary.
II. Title.
RC416.B35A33   1986   362.1′96865   [B]   85-14153
ISBN 0-03-002997-X

First Edition
Designed by Susan Hood
Printed in the United States of America
1   3   5   7   9   10   8   6   4   2

Portions of Bed Number Ten *have appeared in the*
December 1985 issue of Good Housekeeping.

ISBN 0-03-002997-X

The names of the hospital and all medical personnel have been changed to protect those who were less than kind.

This is dedicated to all who cared, so they will know how much they did. And to those who may be called upon to care, so they will know how much they can do.

1

SHUTTING DOWN

1

My toes tingled. Funny. Nothing too unusual. There was no time for concern that Monday morning of December 1, 1980. I had to get moving. I was in charge of the volunteer mothers at my daughter Elizabeth's high school, and this was my day to be on duty.

As Bill shaved, I brushed my hair and slipped on my robe before going down to make breakfast. What could make my toes tingle? Certainly nothing to worry about, I assured myself.

Halfway down the stairs I met Elizabeth, who was still carrying a cup of coffee as she hurried upstairs to dress for school. This was the synchronized routine we'd fallen into—very comfortable for our early-morning schedules. In the kitchen, I removed the orange-juice pitcher from the refrigerator and poured a glass for Bill and then one for me. From the cupboard I removed bowls and our usual box of cereal. Then the bread went into the toaster. As I watched the coils of the toaster turn red, I reached for the first sip of my juice, all in the easy rhythm of habit.

I was startled when I tasted the orange juice. It burned my tongue—and my lips. How odd. I knew it was fresh. The toast popped up and I buttered it. Again the rhythm took over as I carried the bowls, the cereal and milk, the toast, and Bill's juice to the table. I took another drink of orange juice. Again the burning sensation. It had to be my imagination; I'd mixed that juice just last night. It had to be all right. I finished the contents in a single gulp as I looked at the clock. Ten minutes to seven, right on schedule. I walked toward the front of the house just as Elizabeth came down the stairs, ready for her car pool. With a quick kiss on my cheek, she hurried out the door to the waiting car. "Have a good day," I called to her. And, as always, I stood at the door for a moment to wave good-bye. I loved watching her with her friends—all that happy enthusiasm. I closed the door just as Bill came down the stairs, and we walked back to the breakfast table.

I watched Bill's face as he drank his juice. "Is it all right?" I asked. He glanced at me, puzzled, so I added, "It seemed to burn my tongue and lips when I drank mine."

Bill looked at his glass and then at me. "Mine's OK. Tastes fine." I said nothing but decided to try my cereal. It tasted normal. I was relieved.

Silently, I ate my toast, aware that Bill was looking at me occasionally with his are-you-all-right expression. Neither of us said anything, but of course, I *was* all right. Perhaps I had imagined the burning orange juice. I felt the tingling in my toes again, and maybe in my fingers, too. But I said nothing.

Bill finished his breakfast and got up to leave. I followed him out the back door and watched him back the car out of the garage and down the long driveway. It seemed important today that everything be normal, just like always. As he maneuvered onto the street, I waved, savoring just for a moment his returning wave. I wished it weren't Monday. Today especially, what with the long Thanksgiving weekend just finished, I wondered why I'd ever volunteered for Mondays.

It was five after seven when I glanced at the clock. No time for lingering. I hurried back into the kitchen, gathered up our dishes and put them into the dishwasher, then ran upstairs to dress.

As I checked the mirror one last time, I remembered the invitations. Mustn't forget those, I told myself. While Katherine had been home from Vanderbilt over Thanksgiving, she, Elizabeth, and I made out the guest list and addressed sixty-five invitations for their annual holiday buffet. The anticipation of entertaining all their friends made planning this event special to the girls, and doubly so for me. Since this was Katherine's first year away from home—way up in Nashville—we had to do all the planning while she was home. We discussed the details, and Elizabeth and I even set aside all the recipes for the menu. On my way past the desk, I remembered to gather up the stack of invitations.

Houston's morning air was balmy as I walked to the garage. When I put my foot on the car accelerator, the tingling was still there.

The gas gauge was low, so I decided to stop and have the tank filled before going on to the school. Tony was standing beside the pumps as I drove in. Just seeing him was brightening this morning. He had tended our cars for years and was always pleasant. "Hi. How're you doin'?" he asked. Of course I told him I was fine and inquired about his Thanksgiving. I could hear him talking in his usual chatty manner, but it was hard for me to concentrate. He asked if Katherine had come home. I nodded and smiled, rubbing my fingers absently, trying to stop the tingling. And I wiggled my toes.

He took my credit card and wrote up the charge. As I signed the charge slip, the pen felt a little awkward in my hand. Funny, I thought. "You have a nice day now," Tony said with his customary pleasantness. I forced a smile and nodded as I started up the car and drove away, waving my good-bye.

Houston's morning-rush-hour traffic is always distracting, but this morning I welcomed the distraction. I should have turned onto the street that passed the post office and mailed the invitations, but I decided against it. I don't feel like stopping this morning, I thought, surprising myself with the uncustomary procrastination. But I was not feeling just right, so I drove on. I straightened the pile of envelopes and assured myself I would mail them on the way home from the school.

Traffic was picking up, but today I was thankful for all the cars. It was good having people around. This was the route used by many of the students and faculty who lived in our neighborhood. I glanced at other drivers, searching for someone I knew. A familiar face would be reassuring. But all the cars were driven by strangers.

The parking lot of Robert E. Lee High School was half-filled with teachers' and students' cars as I drove in, but no one was arriving at just this moment. I looked at my watch. Seven-forty-five. I was right on time. I liked being ahead of the student rush. As I walked the long hall toward the main office, the corridor seemed darker than usual, although the lights were all on. And the hall appeared so much longer. I could hear voices, somewhat muffled, but the building felt empty.

It was a relief to walk into the familiar main office. At least there were people, voices of welcome.

"Hi, Sue. How was your weekend?" one asked. Another wondered if Katherine had come home. Everyone knew both girls. Elizabeth was still in their midst, and they often asked about their recent graduate, Katherine. My answers were pleasant, a bit forced, almost announcements: It had been a very special holiday; Katherine was fine; she loved Vanderbilt; we were all happy to have the nice, long weekend together.

I was relieved when I could finally sit down at the desk reserved for volunteers and search for my name tag in the file box. I struggled with the clip. Awkward gadget. It just didn't want to go on right today. Faculty members hurried in and out of the office, signing in and then rushing off to homerooms. I smiled at each of them—they had become my friends over the years. But I was grateful this morning that they were all too rushed for conversation. Students came and went. Thank goodness the secretaries were at the counter and able to keep up with their requests. I glanced toward the window; it had started to rain. Suddenly I felt so tired, weak. Nothing specific, just general weakness. Perhaps it was the weather—or the weekend was catching up with me.

My job was to take all incoming calls. I hoped it would be a light morning. Class bells rang; activity moved away from the front counter; chaos subsided. I wasn't the only one breathing a sigh of relief. But the morning rush usually stimulated me, rather than wearing me out. The tingling in my toes had become noticeably more persistent. And in my fingers. Still, there wasn't much time for dwelling on such irritations. The phone kept up a steady ring—calls to transfer, informational inquiries, messages to note. Writing became more difficult. I shouldn't be so tired, I kept telling myself. I had slept well enough the night before.

By ten o'clock I had been able to ignore how I felt. Then came a call for one of the teachers. She would be on break in the faculty lounge, probably waiting for the call. Forcing myself to my feet, I trudged down the hall to the lounge. I stood back to allow her to run on ahead to answer the waiting phone call. As I turned to walk back to the office, I knew for sure that something was wrong with me.

With real effort now, I forced myself back to the office and my desk. Wanda, a secretary in the principal's office, brought me a cup of coffee, as she always did at this time of morning. The expression on my face must have given me away. I tried not to alarm her, but I was not succeeding. I needed more than a cup of coffee this morning.

My mind raced for the name of a doctor. We didn't have a family physician—just the pediatrician who had cared for both girls and continued taking care of all four of us. She was like a member of our family. But no, not for this. Then there was my gynecologist. . . . But today I needed someone else. Finally I thought of my mother's internist, Dr. Lohmann. His office was nearby and at least he knew me, having seen me so often with Mother.

I called Bill and was relieved when he answered the phone. He might have been out of the office. "I'm sorry to bother you, but I feel like something is wrong with me. I need to see a doctor."

He seemed to understand that it was serious. Otherwise, I wouldn't have disturbed him. Within minutes Bill pulled up in front of the school. He had called Dr. Lohmann, who agreed to see me immediately. I was relieved just to see Bill. Wanda insisted on walking me to the door and then partway down the steps until Bill reached me and helped me the rest of the way down and into the car.

I remembered Dr. Lohmann as being kind and sensitive with Mother, and again I felt relief. He saw me immediately and examined me thoroughly, especially testing my reflexes. Everything checked out as normal. He was puzzled. My toes and fingers still tingled, and a slight weakness now affected my walking. And then there was that overall feeling that something wasn't right. I couldn't put a finger on it, or even describe it to the doctor. Bill mentioned that I'd had an intestinal virus the week before. That finally gave Dr. Lohmann a clue. Perhaps, he concluded, it was dehydration or an imbalance of electrolytes.

"You just go home," he said, "and rest and drink lots of Gatorade. And eat bananas." Awful, I thought. I don't like Gatorade! "And if things aren't better by Thursday, we'll do some blood work."

Bill helped me back into the car. I felt unsatisfied without solid answers and wished it would all go away.

My mother lived close by, so I went to her apartment to spend the afternoon, rather than have Bill drive me all the way home. Bill could get back to the office easily and pick me up on his way home from work. Of course, Mother was distressed at my not feeling well, but I assured her I was just fine—merely suffering a little carryover from the flu. If only I could convince myself. We distracted ourselves with talk of the past weekend. Mother had been with us for Thanksgiving day and she was most anxious to hear all about the remainder of Katherine's visit. I loved the telling nearly as much as she enjoyed hearing about it.

I called the school and left a message for Elizabeth to take my car home—and to be sure to drop the party invitations at the post office. Then I rested, just as the doctor ordered.

That night Bill and Elizabeth decided to make dinner. They urged me to continue resting, but it was hard to stay away from the kitchen, so I elected myself supervisor. The evening passed quickly. Normally. Dinner, schoolwork for Elizabeth, and television and reading the evening paper for Bill and me. Then bed. I had no difficulty negotiating the stairs, though the bed was most welcome. I lay there waiting for Bill, staring at the ceiling, hoping I would wake up the next morning and be fine. All the tingling would be gone, I was sure. My weekly 7:30 A.M. tennis game with Janice was set for tomorrow. That would get me back into shape again, I decided. Sleep came easily.

Bill's alarm emitted its early-morning call. Sleepily, I shuffled to the bathroom for my customary first-thing drink of water. The shock jolted me fully awake. I couldn't swallow!

2

I was standing at the closet door, trying to concentrate on what to wear. I could hear Bill talking on the phone to Dr. Lohmann. "Yes," he was saying, "we can be there in an hour or better." I tried to turn my attention back to the closet.

"He'll meet us at Gulfland Hospital, Sue." Bill was standing beside me now. I nodded, not wanting to look at his face and see that apprehensive expression.

"I can't decide what to wear," I said. I felt silly after I let go of the words.

"Just put on anything. It doesn't matter." He was not being harsh, but concern put an extra edge on his voice.

"Bill, please, just go downstairs and fix yourself a piece of toast while I get dressed."

He turned and walked to the door, muttering, "I told him we'd be there in an hour." I understand, Bill! And the traffic will be slow, too. I understand. I focused in on the closet and chose a jeans skirt, a plaid blouse, and my penny-loafers.

At the mirror I again tried to swallow. Nothing. Fear was gripping me, but I forced my attention to the image in the mirror and carefully applied full makeup.

It occurred to me that Dr. Lohmann probably would put me in the hospital overnight for some tests, so I removed a small overnight case from the closet. What do I need for one night in the hospital? I wondered. It had been a long time since I'd had to do this.

Bill returned to the bedroom as I packed. "Don't worry. If you forget anything, I can bring it to you." His words jarred my mental checklist and I suddenly remembered the date. It was past the first of the month.

"My goodness, it's time to pay bills," I said. "I missed yesterday. I'll have to do it today." I sent Bill to get the checkbook and the stack of bills. While he was gone, I remembered my tennis game with Janice. Calling her was his next assignment. Finally I latched the small bag and stood back for Bill to take it. At the bedroom door, I turned back again. The room was warm and comfortable. I felt a sudden sadness at having to leave. I just didn't seem ready.

Surely it couldn't have been a premonition that I would not see this room again for some eleven months.

It was nine o'clock when we arrived at the hospital. Dr. Lohmann had arranged for me to be admitted immediately. We gave the admitting clerk the customary information, and she handed me the form to sign. My hand held the pen poised to write, but I couldn't sign my name. Once again the fear surfaced. I handed the pen to Bill. What's happening to me, I pleaded silently. What's happening to my body? The only response was the clattering noises of a workman down the hallway, mocking my questions.

An attendant brought a wheelchair. I wanted to walk up to the room but was persuaded to accept the ride. Even though my mother had been a patient here, today everything seemed strange. On the way to the elevator, I saw a nurse who worked for an orthopedist we had used over the years. A familiar face! I felt a flutter of excitement. At least there was one familiar face at the hospital now.

Nurses and technicians swarmed into my room. I was measured and weighed. Thermometers, blood-pressure cuffs, syringes drawing blood. Then, as suddenly as it began, it ended, and the room was quiet. Bill and I smiled at one another reassuringly, but there was nothing to say. I was thankful that there was no one in the other bed. It gave us the privacy of a single room. We checked out the accommodations—closets, plumbing, the view from the window—perhaps trying to sound more like seasoned apartment hunters than a frightened patient and a worried spouse.

I was becoming aware of a general feeling of weakness and

fatigue, so I slipped into my pajamas and lay on the bed. Even a hospital bed felt good at that moment. I knew I couldn't sleep, but it was a relief just to close my eyes for a few minutes. Bill alternately sat reading a magazine, paced into the hallway and back, and looked out of the window. I wanted to be home again.

I was sitting up in bed when Dr. Lohmann finally arrived at eleven. He had been waiting for the lab reports. "Well, the blood work is clear," he said. He seemed to be speaking to Bill, rather than to me. "I gave Sue a physical examination yesterday, and she checked out fine. And now we have no clues from today's lab work. I can do nothing else for her, so I am calling in a neurologist." I tried to comprehend his words. What did he mean, he couldn't do anything else for me? "Dr. Muenkel will be in later today to see her. He's a top neurologist, and I'm sure he will be able to find the answers for you." Abruptly he left.

Bill and I sat in silence. I wanted to say, "I truly am sick. I am. Something is really wrong." But I was sure Bill knew that even without my saying anything.

A nurse brought in a tray of soft foods. I was hungry, but still I could not swallow.

Throughout the afternoon, their efforts to get me to eat continued. Juices, gelatin, ice cream. It was useless; nothing would go down. They told me I needed fluids, but I already knew that. Why couldn't I swallow?

Partly to provide distraction, I attacked the pile of bills. The family finances had always been my responsibility, and I was fastidious about the assignment. But now I couldn't write. I turned the ledger-style checkbook over to Bill, explaining each statement to him so he could write the checks and total the balance. I made a point of telling him the details of each account and other things he should know, such as when mortgage payments were due, as well as all the other family business. Making sure he understood everything became a compulsion. I sensed I had to inform him about all of it today.

Occasionally one of us would note the time. Still no Dr. Muenkel. When was he coming? It was so frustrating. Sometimes I wondered if I were merely imagining all that I could feel going on in my body. The increasing weakness, the numbness attacking my feet and hands, my inability to swallow. But the symptoms were so frightening that I knew they were real. And because it was happening to me, I felt that this was an emergency, that I needed medical attention. But still no Dr. Muenkel—or any other doctor.

I told Bill about my schedule for the week. Tomorrow was the monthly meeting of my literature club. I was president, and the vice president had to be notified that I could not be there. Then there was the recommendation letter to write for a prospective member, listing her qualifications to join the group. I dictated from notes I'd remembered to bring along, and Bill wrote out the letter. This, I instructed him, must be dropped off at the vice president's home, along with the gavel and the members' name tags. It was part of my position, and I felt very responsible that it all be done. Of course, Bill agreed.

Also, I had made a luncheon date for Friday. Bill would have to call Bess and cancel that. All of these instructions were carefully noted in Bill's diary. He had carried a small daily logbook in his pocket for years. Each month he replaced it with a new one and filed the old one in his desk drawer. He recorded everything of significance throughout the day in the appropriate hourly time slot. These notes had always been an important part of Bill's research work, and over the years, he had extended the notations to cover his personal life as well. When Dr. Lohmann left, Bill instinctively reached for his diary and entered the basic information. Now he was listing more of my instructions, and it was comforting for me to watch him write—and to know that everything would be accomplished.

In spite of not being able to consume food or fluids, I found myself needing to make frequent trips to the bathroom. Nerves, I presumed. As the afternoon wore on, the need arose more often, and I became weaker with each trip. Eventually, Bill had to help me walk, then to lower me onto the seat and lift me up again. Despite our years together, it was humiliating to need this kind of help from my husband. Neither of us should have to go through this.

Still no Dr. Muenkel. Nothing but occasional visits from the nursing staff. The dinner tray came and had to be returned untouched. Bill continued to write in his diary, listing phone numbers of people he should call if I was required to stay any length of time in the hospital, reminding himself of things to do: to call Katherine, to have some repairs done on the car, to change the cat's litter box.

It was seven o'clock when Dr. Muenkel finally arrived. Now, surely, we would get answers. He checked my reflexes, which he said were good. And he did some pinpricking—without comment. "Well," he began, "at this point I can only tell you that it is probably one of three things." He stopped for a deep breath, more of a sigh. I was sure he could hear my heart pounding. "It could be multiple sclerosis, myasthenia gravis, or Guillain-Barré syndrome. I think we can quite safely rule out myasthenia gravis at this point." All three sounded frightening. "We'll just have to wait until we do a spinal tap tomorrow, and then we'll know." Tomorrow! The words stung me with alarm. "I'm sorry, but that's about all I can tell you at this point."

Panic was overpowering me, but I forced myself to ask calmly about the diseases he had just suggested. Dr. Muenkel smiled, trying to comfort me. "Well, let's just wait until we see what we have before worrying about that." As he spoke, he moved toward the door and then bid us good night. He left before we could ask anything more. But it didn't seem to matter just then. What questions could we have asked? I was consumed by disappointment and fear of the unknown.

Bill and I stared off in different directions. I grappled with the names Dr. Muenkel had mentioned, repeating the words to myself. They all sounded terrifying. The hospital room had become cold and stark. I looked out into the night and yearned to go home. Oh, God, I want to go home! Bill was writing in his pocket diary. I could well imagine what he was writing: Dr. Muenkel says it's M.S. or Guillain-Barré. Probably not myasthenia gravis.

"How do you spell Guillain-Barré?" I asked—more for something to say than for a desire for information.

"I can only guess." Bill put the diary back in his pocket and came over to the bed. He held me, and we both fought back tears. "It'll be all right, Sue. I know it will." I struggled to believe Bill and to draw from him the strength he always gave me.

Soon after Dr. Muenkel left, a young man appeared, identifying himself as James from respiratory therapy. I didn't know why he was here, but there was something about his manner that put me at ease for the first time in this long, torturous day. He explained only that he wanted to take some measurements, so Bill helped me stand beside the bed, and James measured my breathing capacity. It was actually a comfort to have someone doing something about whatever my illness was.

The evening wore on into nighttime. I wanted to send Bill home so he could rest; he looked so tired and strained. He had missed work today, and I knew that he'd have to do twice as much tomorrow to catch up. But I was afraid to have him leave. Thank goodness, we were at a hospital located between home and his office, rather than downtown or at the medical center. At least here he could arrange quick visits to see me on his way home from work. Such a small consolation became important.

At ten-thirty the head nurse came into the room. She looked at Bill, and I was sure she was going to tell him to go. Her voice was measured. "I think, Mr. Baier, that we had better take your wife to ICU."

"Intensive care!" I could hardly speak. "No, I don't need intensive care." Terrified, I looked from the nurse to Bill for concurrence.

"Why?" Bill asked her.

I could hear the nurse speaking as she answered Bill, but the words swirled incoherently. Tell her, Bill, that I must stay here, in this room, until the spinal tap in the morning. Then I'll be going home.

Bill came to my side and spoke softly, gently. "I think you'd better go, Sue."

"No, I don't want to. If I go there, you can't stay with me."

His voice was barely a whisper. "You have to, Sue." His eyes looked sadly into mine. "You haven't been able to eat or drink all day. You know you're getting weaker. I can't leave you like this. You must go so they can take care of you."

The nurse left briefly and returned with a wheelchair. A huge, hard mass formed in my stomach as we packed up my things. Then we were on our way through the blur of now-quiet halls, down in the elevator, and into a long corridor, filled with foreboding.

Bill held open the door as the nurse pushed my wheelchair into the intensive care unit. While she handed my chart to an ICU nurse, I looked around the room. It was even more frightening than I had imagined. There were a dozen or so beds in small, partitioned, three-sided cubicles along the outside walls of a large room. The fourth side of each cubicle opened into the main room, where the nursing station was located. Most of the beds were occupied with patients wired to all manner of machinery and bottles. I recoiled at the sight and let my gaze fall to the floor. But I couldn't shut out the wheezing sounds of respirators. I wanted to run, but I knew I wasn't able to walk, let alone run. I prayed to be gone from this place. Instead, I was wheeled toward a bed. Printed on the back wall behind it was the number ten.

I was welcomed to Bed Number Ten by a young man who introduced himself as Bruce. "I'll be your nurse for the rest of this shift. I hope you find this bed satisfactory," he said as he helped me onto the bed. "According to your chart, you'll probably be with us for at least three months."

I was too stunned to respond. What was he saying? Three months? Horror churned my stomach. No, that could not be. He had to be wrong. I couldn't stay here in this awful place for three months. Besides, Christmas was coming. I had too many things to do. I can't be in a hospital. Not now. Not here.

I was still sitting on the side of the bed, battling with my thoughts, when I was handed a hospital gown. "You'll have to wear a gown in here," Bruce said. "You can put it on now, if you don't mind." I do mind, I thought. I mind very much. Drawing a curtain across the open end of my cubicle, he walked out toward the nursing station, where Bill was waiting. I could hear him telling Bill, "You can take home her pajamas and everything else. All she'll need here is her toothbrush."

As I struggled into the gown, I began to notice a steady drainage from my nose. When Bruce returned, I asked him for some tissues, which he handed me. He reached toward a cart behind him for some kind of apparatus attached to a plastic tube, told me to lie down, and then pushed the tube down my throat. I gagged. Immediately he pulled it out again. "Get used to that because you're going to have a lot of that while you're here."

When I got my breath back, I asked him what he had done. "Nothing, yet," he replied. "I just want you to know what we'll be doing when your condition gets worse."

This can't really be happening, I thought. It has to be a nightmare. But when the curtain was pulled back and Bill was allowed to return to my bedside, I realized it wasn't. His face looked so sad and frightened as he grasped my hand, trying to give me courage. Bruce was there again, telling me I had to take off my rings.

"No, please," I begged. "Not my wedding ring. I've never taken it off. Can't you just tape it to my hand?"

"No. It has to go," Bruce answered flatly.

I fought tears as I tugged to pull off the engagement and wedding rings. My fingers were almost nonfunctioning, but the anger made them work. I could not look at my husband when I handed him the rings. As Bill gathered up my pajamas and robe, Bruce gave him a paper bag to put them into and then asked him to leave.

I was terrified, so frightened of letting go of Bill. He was security. Everything else seemed so abrupt, so unreal. I clung to his hand. We were both trying to be strong. I was not succeeding. Finally, I knew I had to let go, and I watched Bill gather up my case and the paper bag. He kissed me—the way one does at a train station or airport. This was too public a place for either of us. He took only a few steps, then turned back just before he moved out of sight. One last look and then he was gone. Utter despair; total abandonment. Everything in the world was gone with him.

Only Bruce was still there. Plus the wheezing machines, and the dozen pallid patients I could not see but remembered all too vividly. And other nurses whom I did not know, including the new shift that was just coming on duty. Even worse than the tears, my nose was now discharging uncontrollably. I apologized to Bruce for using so many tissues.

3

"December 3: Guillain-Barré confirmed. 6 P.M. respirator."
—from Bill's diary

The clock on the wall opposite my bed stared back its silent message: six o'clock. Was it morning or night? Did it matter? Yes, it did. It must be morning. Six in the morning was a time for getting up, for things to happen. For me to make them happen. I quickly glanced around the room. Nothing had changed. I was still in this miserable place, intensive care. My nose had stopped dribbling, but now saliva was running out of the sides of my mouth. As I turned my head slightly to the side, it gushed from my mouth, down the side of my face and neck, onto the bed. I shuddered with revulsion as I tried to swab away the mess. My hands would not work, but with the little strength left in my arms, I stuffed a tissue into the offensive area. I wanted to call for help but was too embarrassed. I wasn't even sure I still had a voice. The entire unit echoed the sounds of voices, of the clattering of metallic equipment that I could not see. Nor did I wish to.

A night-shift nurse, Gwenn, came alongside the bed, wiped my face, wrapped my fingers around a fresh wad of tissues, and placed my hand next to my mouth. I apologized weakly for using so many—and for the mess. It was humiliating. Although Gwenn had appeared several times during the night, she usually seemed totally baffled about what to do for me. I was sure she would rather I were unconscious. She wouldn't have to talk to a comatose patient, and Gwenn left no doubt in my mind that she preferred not having to speak to me. She wasn't unkind. Just aloof, remote.

I studied my tiny room. Already I thought of it as my room, even though the staff referred to it simply as Number Ten. I didn't want to be here and did not plan to stay, but while I was here, I needed to define this space as mine—my area. Extending just beyond the foot of the bed on either side of me were walls—about three feet from the right side of the bed, four feet from the left. I could not see much of the third wall behind my bed, except to make out the number over my head. The fourth side, at my feet, was open to the nursing station, the hub of the intensive care unit. On each side wall was a large glass window that opened into the next cubicle. On my right, a full-length curtain was drawn across the window and to the end of the wall. I caught only glimpses of the corner of that window as nurses swished past the curtain, and it moved with them. This was the curtain that Bruce had pulled around the open side at the foot of my bed while I put on my hospital gown last night.

To my left, a curtain was drawn across the window from inside the next compartment. I wished that there were a curtain on my side of the wall, too. The fact that someone else had control over uncovering that window left me feeling vulnerable. During the night I had heard the patient in that bed—was that Number Nine or Number Eleven?—being referred to as John. I did not like the idea that John could pull back the curtain from my window. Then I remembered hearing John moaning during the night. I supposed that John was not going to be up and around, peering at me, any more than I would be getting up and changing anything. Nevertheless, I tugged awkwardly at the sheet to be sure I was fully covered. These skimpy hospital gowns did not provide much protection for my six-foot-long body.

Nurses moved past my room frequently. I counted three besides Gwenn. But they never stopped, or even looked in at me. Was I the exclusive property of Gwenn? She paused at the foot of the bed every little while and looked at me, but if I said nothing, she did not acknowledge me or inquire if I needed anything. I rarely asked for anything. I didn't want to be a bother.

I studied the curtain next to my bed. It was cream colored, like the walls. At least it looked freshly laundered. There was a brief feeling of security in looking at that curtain. Nothing else here made me feel secure.

Across from the foot of my bed, in the center of the unit, stood the nursing station, a room within the room. The wall facing me, on which hung the large, round clock, radiated with yellow paint, a rather bright citrus shade. There must be a better color, I thought. A large window, like those at my sides, looked into the station. Or, more precisely, looked out from the station. Nurses moved toward the window occasionally, checking their patients.

A few feet to the left of the window was an open door through which I could see desk space for two nurses. Between the door and the window was the clock. Had the hands stopped altogether, or was it really only six-fifteen?

A bright fluorescent panel in the ceiling above the clock illuminated the area. The entire unit was lighted by these panels, spaced periodically between the large, white, acoustical ceiling tiles that all hospitals seem to use. In fact, another light panel hovered directly over my bed, but it was turned off when not needed. The other—between the clock and my cubicle—burned all night.

I stretched to look at a small exterior window over a bed across the room. It was still dark outside. Of course, it would be. This was December, and the days were short. This was December and I could not be in the hospital! I had just barely started doing the Christmas shopping. There was too much to do for me to waste even a day. Besides, I can recuperate at home just as well as here. Then next week I can get the shopping done and the decorating started. Once again the clock distracted me. It was nearing six-thirty. Bill had promised to be here by seven-thirty, just over an hour. Please come soon, Bill. Please hurry.

Fear surged through me as I tried to roll over onto my side. My body did not have enough strength. Gwenn walked past the bed again, so I summoned the courage to ask her for help. Gently, but passively, she turned me and put a fresh wad of tissues beside my mouth. I thanked her and again apologized about the tissues and the mess. My stomach churned. I wished she at least could have smiled. Even she must be finding my mess disgusting. Tears coursed a trail to the upper edges of the tissue wad and were blotted effortlessly.

New voices rang through the unit. The morning shift was

arriving. With one nurse from the night shift, the new group made rounds, standing at the foot of each bed to be familiarized with that patient's condition. When they came to my bed, I listened carefully.

"Probable Guillain-Barré," Gwenn reported with a passiveness that made me feel invisible—or dead. "Lumbar puncture scheduled for seven-thirty." My heart pounded. The spinal tap! I forgot that was coming. Dear God, please help me. I had heard such terrible things about those. The nurse was continuing with all kinds of medical jargon and letter combinations, alphabets that shut out the patient. I wanted to tell her that I couldn't have a spinal tap at seven-thirty because Bill would be here by then. And I had questions to ask. But the group moved on quickly to the next bed. Their voices were abstract now. Alphabets for another patient. But what about me? What was happening to me? What was this Guillain-Barré? And when were they going to give me some miracle medicine to cure it?

Very shortly, a new nurse named Harriet came to my bedside, rolling a small piece of machinery. "That discharge looks miserably uncomfortable for you," she said, sounding sympathetic. She actually looked at me and knew I was alive! "Do you think you can hold this?" She held up a plastic suction apparatus, the kind dentists use. I nodded. Her smile was genuine and most welcome. She hooked up the cord to an electrical outlet, turned on the switch, and put the tube in my mouth. The swizzling sound was startlingly loud as the gadget evacuated the overflowing cavity. I smiled my gratitude. Then she, too, disappeared.

Finally, forever ended and Bill arrived. It was nearly seven-thirty. "Oh, Bill." My tears choked off the weakened voice. His face looked so sad. He was trying to smile, but tears were glistening in his eyes. He kissed me and held me for a long moment. Both of us struggled for control. He reached for a handful of tissues and wiped the tears from my cheeks and the residue of saliva from the sides of my mouth. I felt helpless, yet grateful to have some of the mess cleaned up.

"I got my first set of chores done today." Now he could smile, finally. Tasks can be diverting. "I just dropped off the letter, name tags, and gavel. Everything was just where you said it was."

"And the lunch date?" I, too, was distracted now.

"Yes, I canceled your luncheon. That's all I had time for, but I'll get at the rest as I can at work today. Just don't worry about one thing." He reached for a bag he had laid at the foot of my bed. "I even remembered a radio for you. I was sure you'd want it." Again I could feel the tears crowding my eyes. Dear Bill. Always so thoughtful. I hadn't even asked for it.

Bill set up the radio and adjusted the volume as we discussed which station I would enjoy most. At home I usually tuned the radio to a talk station while I worked around the house. So that was my choice now. We talked about Elizabeth, about his call to Katherine in Nashville. He had assured her that everything was under control. Neither of us wanted to worry her just a week before final exams. I told him about my uneventful morning and my long night. Bill laughed, saying his night had been very short. I pretended to laugh, too, though I felt overwhelming sadness over his having to go through all this.

The minutes passed so quickly, and too soon Bill was telling me it was time to go. They had rules, he explained. Only three visits a day—and only fifteen minutes at a time. As weak as I was, I clung desperately to his hand and begged him not to leave. "It's the rule, Sue. Besides, they say that any longer a visit would only tire you." The rule, the ultimate answer. Always Bill played by the rules. There was no use trying to fight "the rules." Dejectedly, I let my hand drop. "I'll be back at eleven-thirty. I promise." I heard the sadness in his voice and knew he didn't want to leave any more than I wanted him to go. Bitterness evaporated into a melancholy smile.

"I love you," he said as he kissed me.

"I love you, too." My tears washed away the image of him leaving. When I blinked them away, he was gone. Only the clock was still there. Seven forty-two. Three hours and forty-eight minutes until Bill would return.

A flurry of activity accompanied the arrival of Dr. Muenkel. The spinal tap. I looked at the clock, thankful they hadn't come at seven-thirty.

"Now just relax," Dr. Muenkel was saying after wiping my back with alcohol and pressing his fingers along my spine in search of the proper entry point. There was nothing I could do but relax. I had no strength to resist, even if I wanted. The needle slid in effortlessly. Not nearly what I expected. I wondered why everyone said a spinal tap was so painful. I was ready to ask the doctor about Guillain-Barré, but before I could, he patted my hip and told me to rest, and he and the nurses disappeared.

Within minutes, another nurse came in and said, "All right, Sue, now let's raise up."

I struggled to move, then I remembered. "I just had a spinal tap. Don't you get headaches if you get up?"

"Oh, yes," she answered with alarm. "Get back down!" She's supposed to know what's going on here, I thought. She should have known.

Nurses moved toward and away from my bed. I was turned, pillows were propped against my back to keep me from rolling over. Harriet inserted a catheter. Did this mean I was losing bladder control—or, more serious, kidney function? Apprehension mounted anew. Kidney problems were common in my family. She assured me that I need not worry. Now I just wouldn't have to be concerned about elimination. Not much to be concerned about, I wanted to say; I've had nothing to eat or drink for thirty-six hours. I felt all the more helpless. Each time I was turned, I assured everyone that I was comfortable, even when I wasn't. I didn't want to seem troublesome or hard to please.

I could feel myself drifting in and out throughout the morning. The radio droned on. Though I didn't follow the chatter, it was constant and familiar. Dreams slithered into reality. I was in a hospital and Bill was there beside me. "We have our baby girl, Sue. We have our Katherine." We were laughing and crying all at once. Neither of us had cared if we had a boy or a girl. While we waited for our first child, several friends suffered miscarriages and infant deaths. All we wanted was a healthy baby. Bill was still laughing. "And she has exactly ten toes and ten fingers!" The laughter swarmed around me hauntingly.

"Sue . . . Sue." A faceless white blur was shaking me. "Are you awake, Sue?" Now I could see a nurse's uniform. "It's Harriet, and this is Karen." I tried to focus on where I was. Were they bringing Katherine to me? No, they didn't have my baby. Oh, God, please help me. What am I doing here? This is all wrong.

"We need to hook you up with an IV," Karen was saying. "You'll feel more comfortable when you get some fluids into your body."

"And some breakfast," Harriet added. She was smiling genially. "It's all in this little bag." I knew she was trying to add a little humor. I tried to smile in response, but my lips felt as if they'd been injected with Novocain. The nurses turned me to my other side, and as Karen straightened the back pillows, Harriet poked the needle into my arm. I could feel it. I was thankful, at least, for that. I could still feel. I tried to remember all the questions I wanted to ask, but before I could form the words, Harriet and Karen were gone.

The wall clock stared at me, its hands plodding slowly on their course. It was nine fifty-seven. One hour and thirty-three minutes until Bill would come again. The radio droned on. I tried to imagine that I was home, straightening up the family room. The news was about to come on. I must concentrate. Another murder, another fire, three people killed in an automobile accident. Another beautiful day for Houston. But not for Sue Baier. I wanted the announcer to report that. Perhaps he did.

Bill arrived just as the clock's big hand marked eleven-thirty. I tried to reach up to him, but I could not. I wanted to say, "I love you" as he kissed me, but my lips did not want to move. Only guttural sounds emerged from my throat. But he knew. "I love you, too." Again he wiped my cheeks and the sides of my mouth with tissues. The suction tube had fallen from my mouth while I'd dozed and I was unable to replace it. Ever so gently, he sopped up the accumulated pool inside my mouth. I fought tears. He should not have to do this, but I was so thankful that he did. Carefully he returned the suction tube to my mouth and wrapped my fingers around it.

My eyes never left his. There was something there—something dreaded. With the busywork finished, he could avoid it no longer. He looked down and seemed to be studying his hands as he prepared to speak.

"It's Guillain-Barré, Sue." His voice broke as he said my name. Now he could look at me again, and read the anxiety—the unspoken questions. "I don't know much about the disease, Sue. I'm not sure anyone does. They say it's rare." He paused for a deep sigh. "They say you will get well, but . . . but it may be a while." Another painful pause. "You may be here for six weeks . . . or more."

Six weeks—or more? The terrifying prediction of Bruce flashed through my mind. ". . . you'll probably be with us for at least three months." A long, low, horrified "No-o-o-o-o," escaped my worthless lips. And again, "No, no, no, no!"

Bill clasped my free hand so hard that it hurt. His head lowered to rest on our joined hands, as if to emphasize the bonding of our pain. He appeared to be praying. I tried to pray, also, but just then I could only feel my own fear and see Bill's terrible anguish. Finally he straightened up, pulled a handkerchief from his pocket, and wiped his face, staring now at the curtain at the other side of the bed.

He was still looking away. "Dr. Lohmann called me at the office to tell me the diagnosis. He has only seen one other case of Guillain-Barré. He said that one was quite mild. Dr. Muenkel thinks yours may be a little more serious, but he is sure you will be fine." He looked down to see if I was listening. I certainly was. "Remember a few years ago when a lot of people got so sick after taking the swine flu shots?" I nodded. I did remember. "Well, this is what they had." My mind raced, trying to recall what I had heard then. Nothing came back.

"I stopped in to see the company nurse after Dr. Lohmann called. She pulled out a medical book that had a short paragraph on Guillain-Barré." He paused and reached for his notepad. "Let's see. It's an inflammation of the nerves, and it usually follows some other infection, like your intestinal virus." So there was a connection. Bill went on. "Starts in the legs and moves up rather quickly. Usually plateaus for a couple of weeks, and then everything gradually returns to normal again."

He understood when I slurred the words, "Are you sure?"

"Yes, Sue, I am sure." His words were emphatic. "You *are* going to get well." I wanted to ask more, but I wasn't even sure what the questions would be. "We just have to be patient now and let this run its course." His affected acceptance was infuriating.

We have to be patient. I wanted to shout at him. WE! No, it's Sue who has to be patient. I'm the one who is supposed to lie here for six weeks. Six weeks! Or is it to be three months? Again I tried to speak, managing just one heartbroken word: "Christmas!" He understood the word, but ignored my meaning. "You'll be much better by then, Sue. It will all work out fine."

Fear seemed to be drowning me as I tried to deal with this new information. It was overwhelming. "I'm afraid I have stayed longer than my fifteen minutes, Sue. I'd better leave before they kick me out. They have said I can come in at five-thirty, instead of the regular evening visiting time. That way, I can come by on my way home from work." I nodded. "Your mother and Elizabeth want to come in today at five-thirty with me. I think that's good." I didn't want either one of them to see me like this, but they needed to know I was being taken care of. Bill was right. It was best if they came with him. Again I nodded. With a kiss and a wave he was gone—to bury his fears and sorrow in his work. For me there was the clock: eleven forty-eight. Another five hours and forty-two minutes until he returned.

How would Elizabeth and Mother deal with all this? And how would I ever get ready for Christmas now? I concentrated on Christmas. Happy memories, that's what I needed to think about. Perhaps the diagnosis was incorrect. It was probably just a relapse of the flu. I should have taken more time to get over that virus. But now I would get plenty of rest, and within a couple of weeks, at most, I would be back home. Mother and Bill could take care of some of my shopping, but I would be there for the final preparations. This must be our best Christmas ever. I dozed off, mentally hanging ornaments on the trees.

A constant stream of nurses interrupted my tree decorating. I began to receive shots of cortisone. Was this the miracle drug I needed? I was turned from one side to the other. My mouth was suctioned and my face wiped off. Blood pressure and pulse were taken, IV bag was changed. I was thankful when the attending nurse was Harriet. She always chatted so cheerfully. With her, I felt human.

At two-thirty the new shift started wandering in. I could hear them before they were visible. Their hellos announced each new arrival. I didn't want Harriet to leave. Rounds again.

"Confirmed Guillain-Barré. Make sure she's turned every two hours. Monitor respiratory function every hour." Respiratory function? I was breathing fine. Perhaps I was getting a little weaker—a great deal weaker. That's why everything was more difficult, even breathing. But really I was just tired. I heard no more of my report.

The tree trimming resumed. Elizabeth, Katherine, and I. Laughter, home, the smell of fresh pine, Christmas music. Strangers' voices tried to intrude on our special time together, but I shut them out. When the tree was finished, resplendent with its customary pink, white, and gold ribbons, birds, and ornaments, we three turned to Bill for approval. His face was so earnest. "Sue, Sue, I'm here. Elizabeth and Nana are out in the hall waiting to see you." Where had all the pretty ribbons gone? Why was I in this bed, with Bill leaning over me?

The Christmas tree was just a dream; the music vaporized with a flick of a radio switch. I was still imprisoned in the ICU. The immensity of my disappointment must have shown on my face.

"I love you, Sue," he whispered. Concern was vivid in his face. I dared not blink and release the wellspring in my eyes. With great effort I made myself repeat his words of love. He smiled, obviously relieved that I was still conscious. "I'll get Elizabeth and Nana. Try to be in good spirits for them, Sue." He was right. I didn't want to alarm either of them. I would try to think positively.

Elizabeth was a believer, in the fullest sense. It showed in her serene appearance as she walked to my bedside. She assured me that she knew with certainty I would get well, and that confidence radiated from her face. Her smile was warm and genuine. But Mother's face held no secrets from me. Always a woman of strong faith and courage, she was at this moment staggered with shock and horror. As if someone were holding a mirror before me, in her face I saw the full enormity of my illness. She tried to speak through lips frozen by fear and anguish. Then she excused herself on the pretext of wanting Bill to be able to return to my bedside. I watched her shoulders heave with silent, desperate cries of grief as she walked away.

Elizabeth asked the proper questions about how I felt. Was I being cared for properly? Was I comfortable? I nodded affirmative answers. Then, as Bill returned, she asked about the party, the holiday buffet we had planned—and mailed invitations for. "Daddy says we have to cancel it. But I don't want to. I want to have the party. I'll do all the work myself, I promise." The words were pouring out, but Bill interrupted.

"Elizabeth, you know we can't go ahead with that party. It's ridiculous. Your mother is here, very ill, in the hospital."

She continued looking at me. "Mother's going to be fine. We know that. And I can do the party by myself. All the recipes are already set out for the menu. I know I can do it. And Katherine will help me. Please, let us go ahead with the party." Her gaze never left my face.

I glanced away from her, saw Bill's obvious frustration, then looked back to Elizabeth's intense expression of entreaty. I knew how much this yearly event meant to the girls. They would be going through enough with my illness. I couldn't bear the thought of their hurt and disappointment at having to give up their party on my account. Anything either of them had ever set her mind to had been accomplished. Why should I now deny Elizabeth my faith that she could do this on her own? Both of the girls needed this, perhaps more this year than ever. Bill was shaking his head slowly, but firmly, from behind her. Rarely did I countermand Bill's wishes, but now I was sure I was right. With the persistence of youth, Elizabeth asked again, "We can go ahead with the party, can't we, Mother?" I looked at Bill as I responded with a series of slow nods. I watched his jaw tighten, but he said nothing.

Elizabeth was ecstatic. She leaned over and hugged and kissed me and hurried out to the hallway to tell her grandmother. Nana will understand, I told myself. Bill took my hand. "This doesn't make sense, Sue."

Again I forced my tongue and lips to work, however badly. "Yes, it does. Life needs to go on normally, at least for her!" Bill shook his head slowly, wearily. He wanted to protest, but he would not.

At that moment I was startled to see Jo walking toward my bed. She and her husband were good friends from church, yet I knew Bill would not have called her. His surprise at her appearance told me I was correct. She must have heard through church somehow, which meant my condition was considered serious. But surely the message had been exaggerated.

It was wonderful to see her, but immediately I felt embarrassed about how bad I looked—the drooling, the mess on my face and on the bed. My hair had not been combed all day. I always tried to be fastidious about my grooming—not vain, just meticulous. Jo had seen me only at church functions, where I always was dressed most carefully. Now I was too weak even to fluff up my hair.

Jo seemed not to notice. Her voice and her face showed only concern and caring; her words were kind and gentle. She offered encouragement, hope, and the promise of prayers. The suction tube swizzled in my mouth. Her face indicated apprehension. Again embarrassed, I willfully forced words, "Really not as bad as it looks." She left as gently and graciously as she had entered.

Bill checked his watch. Even without looking up at the wall clock, I knew it was time for him to leave. I was tired now, yet it would be nearly fourteen hours until he returned. How could I survive alone here for fourteen hours? Bill's face showed his weariness and anguish, though he struggled to mask both. What a burden I had become for him.

Soon after the family left, two nurses arrived, pulling a cart loaded with equipment and drawing the curtain closed behind them. As they opened packages and rearranged tubes and hoses, they carried on a steady banter of easy chatter, along with asking me *Yes* and *No* questions. Bill was such a fine man. My mother was so attractive. Wasn't Elizabeth a joy? Was I feeling any general discomfort? Didn't I have another daughter? Away at school?

I wondered why they were here. What was coming now? They were so pleasant and courteous, and I was brought up to be polite, so I responded to all their questions. Then came the news. I was going to be hooked up to a respirator. They would place a tube in my nose and down to my lungs to facilitate my breathing. It had to come to this. I was too exhausted to care.

My eyes focused on the clock. Nine-fifteen. I must have slept. What a blessed gift sleep was, but what a cruel disappointment to wake up to all this. A new sound. Of course—the respirator. Now I was just like the other pathetic creatures I'd seen lying in all those other beds. My neck was limp and my head rolled to the side. That slight, involuntary movement dumped an ocean of saliva down my cheek. The thought of it made me cringe with disgust. I tried my voice. No sound.

I was terrified. What was happening? At least I am not dying. Bill had given his promise on that, and he would never lie to me. But was this what living was going to be like now? Was this how I was going to spend the long weeks—or months? Oh, God! All alone? Just machines, tubes, and a fluorescent light glaring in my face. And a clock that would mark the passage of my life silently in this world of no communication. Panic intensified as I realized that now I could not even call for help.

Suddenly Bill appeared at the foot of the bed. Was I dreaming? No, there would never have been tears in Bill's eyes in my dreams. But this was all so frightening that I could no longer separate real from unreal. When he kissed me, I knew for sure; Bill was real. Immediately he grabbed a handful of tissues, wiped off my face, and cleaned out my mouth. His voice was tender and gentle as he spoke of his decision to drop back in to see me. A nurse had called to tell him I was on the respirator. Was the tube terribly uncomfortable? I tried to respond. There was no voice, and my mouth would not move, except for a small twitch to one side. No movement of my head, my hands, or any other part of my body.

"Can you nod your answer, Sue? Is the tube uncomfortable down your throat?"

I am trying, I am trying, I shrieked silently. My eyes widened in terror and frustration. He read the look. "It's all right, Sue. It's all right." He thought a moment. "You're blinking your eyes. Can you blink just once if you're able to control the movement of your eyelids?"

I forced myself to be calm. Then one slow, deliberate blink.

Bill smiled for the first time. "Good. Now, your mouth seems to twitch to one side. Try to move it, and then blink once—*yes*—if you can control that, too." With effort I moved the mouth, not sure if it was even perceptible to Bill. Then I blinked. "Great! The mouth can indicate *no*, and a blink for *yes*. Now . . . is the tube down your throat terribly uncomfortable?"

No, I signaled. Bill smiled, obviously pleased, and clasped my hand. He followed this first success with a series of questions, mostly insignificant—an effort, I was sure, to show me how easily we could communicate. But I had questions, too, and I could not ask them. What if I lost control of my mouth altogether? And my eyelids? What else was going to stop working? Perhaps Bill could read those questions in my eyes, for he sobered as he asked one more question. "Shall we pray together, Sue?"

My response was one emphatic blink.

Cupping his strong, comforting hands around my limp fingers, he bowed his head and prayed silently, pouring a soothing balm over my worst fears. For this brief moment, at least, I felt at peace. Our spirits spoke together, as one, to a Father we trusted to bring us through whatever might lie ahead.

Though Bill could not see it, I smiled at him as he left, and I blew a kiss with my motionless lips and useless hand. We would make it!

Only when the new shift came on duty at eleven, and the expressionless face of Craig stood beside my bed, changing my IV, did the fear return: the terrifying reality that until seven-thirty tomorrow morning, when Bill would return, I was totally at the mercy of people I did not know and with whom I could not communicate. People who didn't even seem to care.

I willed not to think about them. The voices on the radio—they will keep me going tonight. The intravenous bag released its life-sustaining fluid. Drop, drop, drop. It was a rhythm that was syncopated with the wheezing of the respirator. I will *make* it. I *will* make it. I will *make* it.

2
HANGING ON

4

Loud male voices woke me with a jolt. It took an instant for me to realize that the radio station had suddenly come back on the air with the morning farm-and-garden report. The station had signed off during the night, and no one had turned off the radio. As the farm report droned on, I focused on where I was. The reality was shattering.

Although I had been startled awake, nothing moved. In real life, one jumps a little after such a start, but I was unable to move. This could not be real. Yet it was not a dream, either. Throughout the night I had been reminded forcefully that my life was now some new, surreal horror of alternating sleep and wakefulness.

I'd been dozing. I couldn't tell how long. Why hadn't I looked at the clock when I was last awake so I would know how long I'd slept! I was impatient with myself. That was the least I could do—keep track of the time and know how much sleep I was getting. Perhaps it didn't matter; the nights and days of the universe would go on without my timing them.

But not my world. I must not allow myself to lose contact with time. All I could be sure of now was the clock across from my bed. It was four o'clock, and I knew it was morning. That was important. I had to keep in touch with reality, to mark the passage of days and nights.

Today is . . . Wednesday—no, Thursday—December 4. Bridge Club day. I want to go and play bridge today. What am I doing here? Another day closer to Christmas and so much not done. What am I to do about Christmas? Weeks, Bill had said. I don't have weeks to lie here helpless. I have Christmas to prepare for—and Bridge Club.

I felt the tube down my throat; harshly it reminded me of the respirator at the left side of the bed. I was already so accustomed to the noise that for a moment I had not noticed it, but that moment was short-lived. The respirator was there and would not be ignored.

The light over my head went on abruptly. Though I hadn't known a moment of darkness since leaving home, the added brightness hurt my eyes. Craig was standing there, seemingly oblivious of the radio—and of me. He was ready to turn me again. Not a word, not even a glance at my face. Suddenly, I recognized the voices on the radio, and they irritated me beyond reason. This program had been on this station since I was in my teens. In fact, one of the men had been an Extension agent in Fort Bend County, where I grew up. They are a pair of Aggies from Texas A&M and have been joking around for years with typical Aggie stories. When we were first married, Bill and I set our clock radio to wake up to them. But today their patter disturbed me.

I tried to move my lips, just a little twitch of my mouth to indicate *no*. Nothing moved. Crushing disappointment. But it didn't matter to Craig. Methodically he checked my blood pressure and pulse, my vital signs. Craig, I thought, you certainly should have failed your course on bedside manner. Without a word, he rolled me slowly, firmly, to my left side, again propping pillows behind my back. He didn't notice the wetness of my right cheek, or the pool that must have accumulated on the bed, or the new gush that was now coursing down my left cheek. Silently, he turned off my light and disappeared. I was left with the radio and the farm reports.

Through tearful eyes I stared at the respirator. That monstrous machine to which I was wired just kept on pumping. I could not breathe without it. Stifling fear was seizing me. Frantically, yet methodically, I took inventory of every part of my body. Toes: nothing. Legs: no movement, no muscle tensing. My torso knew only the enforced breathing prompted by the respirator. No movement of my body, my neck—nothing. Nor my mouth. Only my eyelids still moved.

Only my eyelids! How would I communicate with Bill? He would be here in three hours. Could it possibly have been seven hours since he left? What were we going to do now? I tried again and again to move my mouth. Everything was gone. My heart pounded with terror. At least it was still beating.

I told myself that this was the way it was going to be temporarily. Remember that, Sue. This is just temporary. But the real terror was surfacing. This disease is rare. Does the staff know how to treat it? Do they know how this feels? I am constantly alone. The nurses are close by in that nursing station, but they are busy talking, laughing, doing other things. I know they have monitors on me, but how can they be so indifferent and cold?

The new shift came on rounds. Craig reported "no change" in my condition. That's not true—my mouth won't move now. If only he'd looked at me, he would have known to report that.

They went on to John's bed. A woman had come to his cubicle during the night. Perhaps it was his wife. She walked away crying, not knowing I was watching her. I wished I could say something to comfort her, but she never even knew I was there.

Promptly at seven-thirty, Bill arrived. His touch was good and familiar. How I wanted to return his sweet kiss. "It's a little cool this morning. A blue-norther coming through." With wads of tissue he cleaned out the mess in my mouth and then wiped off both cheeks. Oh, thank you, Bill.

"Did you sleep well last night?" How do I answer him? Frantically I fluttered my eyelids. "No, Sue, one blink for *yes* or move your mouth for *no*." Oh, Bill, always by the rules. But the rules have changed. Again I blinked repeatedly. He studied me for a moment, and again I blinked my eyes several times. Then he understood. "You can't move your mouth, can you? Is that what you're trying to tell me?"

One firm, elaborate closing and opening of the lids. *Yes*.

"Well, then, how about one blink meaning *yes* and two for *no*?" I blinked once.

"Good. Now, did you sleep well last night?" I blinked once, paused an instant and then blinked again twice. Bill looked puzzled and then suddenly broke into a broad grin as he articulated my message. "*Yes* and *no!*" I responded with one blink.

Now Bill was smiling broadly. "It was the same for me. I was so tired when I hit the pillow, but I kept waking up all night."

Oh, Bill. How upsetting all this must be for you. And how exhausting, having to take care of everything at home as well as to come here.

"I wish I didn't have to run so soon, Sue, but I have a department meeting at eight. I'll be back at eleven-thirty, though. I promise." He turned and looked at the wall clock. "See, less than four hours." Again the kiss and wave, and he was gone. But true to his promise, as Bill always was, he returned exactly at eleven-thirty. Again the warm, tender moment for a kiss, a wad of tissues wiping out my mouth, and another for my face. Then he smiled and rubbed his hands together up and down in a way that told me he had hit upon a splendid idea.

"Your *yes* and *no* answers aren't enough. You can't tell me anything, just answer questions, right?" I wanted to blink a half-dozen times to agree emphatically, but I did just one very exaggerated blink. His smile indicated he understood my emphasis. "All right, let's try one word. Is there one word you can think of that you'd like to tell me?"

Yes. I had no problem choosing the word.

"All right, let's go. The first letter—is it a consonant?" One blink.

"Is it a B?" Two blinks.

"Is it the letter C?" Again two blinks.

On he went, listing consonants until he got to H, and I responded with just one eye movement.

The second letter, I indicated, was not a consonant, so he began with the vowels and proceeded until I responded affirmatively to O. Next we were back to the consonants. Realizing how long it had taken to reach the first letter, he asked, "Is it in the first half of the alphabet?" *No,* I blinked. He began with N and still had a long way to go before reaching T.

Bill was pleased. "Hot! That's it, isn't it, Sue? You're hot?"

Yes! Oh, how warm I was. The respirator spewed out a steady blast of hot air. Even growing up in Texas in the days before air-conditioning, I never adjusted to the heat of summer. And that was exactly what this hot exhaust felt like, just inches away from my bed. Bill felt my forehead and then looked in surprise at his hand. He had wiped off a handful of perspiration.

"Why, you *are* hot. You're covered with perspiration." With another handful of tissues, he wiped my forehead, my face, and then my neck. He finally noticed the covers pulled up under my arm. "Would you like me to take this blanket off you?"

Oh, please, Bill! *Yes*. And the sheet.

Carefully, as if I were fragile and might break, Bill separated the blanket from the sheet and pulled it back, folding it neatly at the foot of the bed. Again he smiled. "There. That's better, isn't it?"

No. It was better, but I wanted that sheet off, too.

"*No?*" He looked at the bed and at my face again. "But you do want the sheet on, surely?"

Two deliberate blinks. *No*. No, please take it off.

He looked around. I could see his frustration. I kept my eyes on him. I intended to hold my ground.

"You don't want the sheet?" There was a note of resignation in his voice.

No.

Slowly he drew down the sheet, carefully lapping the hospital gown and pulling it down to cover as much of me as possible. His expression was definitely dubious as he turned to face me.

"Is that better?" He expected a *no* but got only one blink. Oh, how I wished I could spell *thank you* to him. He could not know how grateful I was.

"I have to get back." I looked at the clock. He'd been here for nearly twenty minutes. A rule broken! "I'll be back at five-thirty." His hand stroked my leg once, ever so gently. I knew how much he hated to leave me "exposed" like this, how reluctant he was to leave without covering me again. But he kissed me, waved, and left.

Now I knew for sure I would make it. I could cope. I could actually *tell* Bill what I needed. And he would make sure that the staff heard me.

I basked in that reality for only a few minutes before Roxann, my shift nurse, came in to check my IV and turn me again. "Oh, Sue," she said as she turned on the light. "You're all uncovered. You must be chilled clear through." As soon as she had me settled on my back, she covered me snugly with both the sheet and the blanket.

Bill and Mother arrived together, exactly at five-thirty. I had been watching the second hand sweep the face of the clock for an hour before they arrived. A look of anguish tugged on the features of Mother's face. While she stood at the foot of the bed to compose herself, Bill came to me with his loving kiss. His hand reached instinctively for tissues to wipe out my mouth.

"Sue, you're soaked with perspiration. And you're all bundled up again with covers. What happened? Did you get a chill?"

No. No chill—just these crazy nurses who insist on covering me from head to toe!

Bill removed the blanket, then loosened the sheet, without removing it. He noticed a washcloth on the nightstand, moistened it in the corner sink, and washed off my face. Oh, how glorious!

Mother stood by, watching quietly, patting my foot almost constantly. Her face relaxed as she watched the activity. "Shall we leave the sheet on for a while, until you dry off?"

No. I was never going to dry off until air could get at my body. Once again, Bill shook his head reluctantly and pulled back the sheet slowly, straightening my gown as he did so.

Mother was totally astonished. "Oh, you can't uncover her like that. She'll catch cold."

Bill was very patient. "She wants the sheet off."

I closed my eyes to shut out the discussion. I knew Bill would handle it.

"Are you awake, dear?" Mother was beside me now, softly brushing the hair back from my forehead with her hand. How often she had soothed me as a child with that hand to my forehead. I blinked once as I looked into her sad eyes, wishing, as I was sure she did, that she could make all this go away with that tender gesture.

"See, Ruth, she blinked *yes*," Bill said from the background.

"Oh . . . yes, she did, didn't she?"

There was an awkward pause as Mother braced herself to speak again. "I had Bridge Club today, Sue." Yes, I'd remembered this was our meeting day. "It just didn't seem right without you. But it really would have been difficult to cancel on such short notice. This way I just called Margie to fill in. Then I could tell them all together that you were here." She was speaking quickly now, obviously having mixed feelings about playing bridge without me. But there was no reason for that. Just because I was in the hospital that didn't mean everyone else's life had to stop.

Mother had been a member of my bridge group for several years. Bridge is something we enjoy together. When Mother had a hip replacement and then eye surgery, she stayed with us to recuperate. On both occasions, my turn came to entertain my two-table club and someone couldn't come. So it was very natural to ask Mother to substitute. It gave her a social outlet. The next month, someone else asked her to fill in. It pleased me that all my friends really liked Mother and enjoyed her company. By the end of the season, Mother was back in her apartment, ready to entertain on her own. So she said, "You've all been so nice to invite me. May I have you one time?" She fixed a lovely lunch for us, and that day the group unanimously agreed to make Mother a regular member of the club. Today had been her turn, and I knew she'd been planning for the group all week.

"I hope you don't mind, dear, that we went on without you today?"

No. Of course, I didn't mind.

"There, Ruth, she's saying *no* by blinking twice," Bill explained. For a moment, Mother seemed relieved and actually forced a smile. But then she looked down at my long, bare legs and the look of dismay returned. Slowly she turned and moved toward the foot of the bed, again patting my feet. I blinked rapidly at Bill. "You want to say something, Sue?"

Yes. Mother looked back, curious. Bill began the laborious process, struggling until he got the word, *win.*

"Win? Oh, the bridge game. Ruth, I think she wants to know who won today. Right, Sue?"

Yes. For the first time, Mother smiled openly. I was greatly relieved.

"Margie did. She made a small slam the last hand, complete with 150 honors. No one else came near." This was more like Mother. As she spoke, she moved back to my side. "Everyone sends their love, Sue. You'll be hearing from all of them soon, I'm sure." I blinked once, slowly. "Bill, did you see that? She does understand." Bill smiled at Mother's delighted surprise. But he was also looking at his watch. How quickly the fifteen-minute visit passes. Mother knew, too, and stepped back to allow Bill to return to my side.

"How are we going to get these nurses to leave the covers off you, Sue?" Again we spelled.

Joan.

"Joan? Is that your nurse?" One blink. "You want me to tell Joan to leave the covers off tonight. All right. That we can do."

While he stepped out toward the nurses' station in search of Joan, Mother came back to say good night. As she leaned over to kiss me, her hand never stopped patting me. She was fighting back the tears. Poor Mother. She'd been through so much this past year. Daddy had been in a nursing home for four years before he died just last spring. She shouldn't have to be worrying about me now.

Bill returned with the news: Joan would leave the covers off, so I could relax now. As Bill leaned over to kiss me, I mentally threw my arms around him for a good hug. How blessed I am to have you, dear Bill. I love you. We spoke the words simultaneously. I wished he could have heard mine.

As soon as Bill and Mother left, Joan appeared. "What's this I hear about your not wanting any covers?"

Yes, I blinked.

"Oh, yes. That nice husband of yours told me about the blinking. That was one for *yes,* I believe." She smiled. "Does that mean, 'Yes, I want covers'?"

I shot back a firm *no*.

She was smiling broadly. "My, that was a strong response. Those eyes were flashing. Don't worry, Sue. I won't cover you— not until you want me to." She took my vitals silently. "Everything looks good. Your husband . . . Bill, isn't it? . . ."

Yes.

"He's a fine man. You're very lucky to have him." She smiled as I blinked agreement. "Ah, that's a very different look this time." Gently, this petite brunette rolled me over to the other side, walked around the bed, and tugged the undersheet smooth. She removed a wrinkle that had plagued me all day. What a relief! Carefully, she positioned my feet and legs, then my free arm. "How's that? Are you comfortable?"

Yes. Thank you, Joan, thank you very much.

I fell into a deep, wonderful sleep. I was playing cards with my group again. But the cards had no printing on them. I knew I had one king and three queens, but there were no faces. My friends were all at other tables; my partner and two opponents were strangers. I bid a grand slam and I had no aces. I should have played the hand, but instead, I was the dummy, so I didn't know what cards my partner had. And I couldn't remember what was trump. He was leading, and always our opponents' cards were higher, but we were taking trick after trick. That was changing the rules! "How lucky you are," Mother kept saying from another table. "How lucky you are."

During the hours that followed, I partially awoke every time Joan came to check me. She always asked me some question. Was I comfortable? Was I warm enough? Each time I answered, she was pleased. So was I.

Finally, the new shift was making rounds. Already I knew the procedure. The party was led by whichever nurse was in charge of the outgoing shift. Joan made her report on me, and though her voice was so soft I couldn't hear what she said, I was sure she told them to leave the covers off.

I was concerned about who would be my nurse for the next shift. I saw Craig and Bruce and prayed it would not be either of them. It was such a relief when a new person announced she would be my nurse. She was an attractive brunette and seemed friendly.

Linda was pleasant and thoughtful as she took my vitals and turned and positioned me. "Joan said you didn't want to be covered, but your feet are cold. I'm sure you'll want covers tonight. It will be getting cooler in here." Slowly, without even looking at my face, she drew up first the sheet and then the blanket, tucking in everything securely on each side.

She turned off the light, saying, "See you later, Sue. Good night." I silently shouted my protest. But she neither heard nor saw.

5

"December 7: Lohmann says fever to be expected. Shell party."
—from Bill's diary

The days and nights dragged on. I made my mind focus on the clock, on the shifts. Staff kept changing. Doctors, nurses, and respiratory therapists came and went with each shift. I alone was trapped here. Except for my eyelids, every part of me had shut down. Entombed in my immobile body, I could see the tiny universe of intensive care. I was a spectator, watching a world that never stopped moving. Through it all, Bill arrived unfailingly.

"Do you want me to uncover you, Sue?" Bill asked when he and Elizabeth arrived in late morning.

No. I couldn't understand why, but the cover felt good. Quite a change, I thought.

"I figured that. You're not perspiring today." Like a solicitous parent, he felt my forehead. "You're running a little fever. That's why you may feel chilled at times."

How was I to spell *how high*, when it was such an effort?

"You're getting antibiotics, shots, and it should be down by tomorrow, so don't worry." That explained the shots I was getting in my hip every four hours. Why didn't the staff tell me why I needed them?

This was Sunday. Bill had not come in early because of church, and now he was telling me about the services. It didn't seem right, my not being able to go to church with Elizabeth and him. We had been members at St. Philip Presbyterian since the girls were in elementary school. Bill was an elder, and very involved in church activities.

"Everyone's praying for you, Sue. The whole congregation." His sentences seemed slow and sad. Elizabeth nodded her agreement. "It was hard walking into church without you this morning. It just didn't seem right. But Sam announced your illness from the pulpit, and everyone prayed for you." Sam Lanham was our pastor, and Bill, as elder, worked closely with him. I was thankful, both for the prayers and for the comfort they gave Bill and Elizabeth. "After services, everyone stopped us and sent their love and best wishes." Bill drew a handkerchief from his pocket and wiped his eyes. "They're all pulling for you, Sue."

I felt their love—its gentle, healing warmth. I was so grateful for what their support meant to Bill right now.

Elizabeth talked of school and clubs. She was involved in so many activities. I'd always known what she was doing, and now I missed the after-school reports on her activities. But we agreed she would come mostly on weekends. I didn't want her missing out on important things in school. Now I listened eagerly, and she seemed as anxious to tell me as I was to hear. Listening to her, I almost imagined I was home again, getting her news.

Suddenly I realized that this was the day of the company party. I had so looked forward to it. This was the first year we had been invited, and I'd been in the midst of making a dress for it when I fell ill. In fact, just before I got sick, I had been feeling very industrious and cut out a wool suit, two blouses, a wool dress, and, especially for this party, a green silk crepe dress. Now all that fabric lay in a pile near the sewing machine at home. The party would have to go on without me tonight, and without my green silk dress.

But not without Bill. I insisted he go. I felt he needed to do something that was not related to the hospital. And I wanted him to tell me about the party.

"No way," Bill said. "This is no time for a party." I understood his not wanting to go alone, especially under the circumstances. But these were people he knew and felt comfortable with at work. And I wanted some contact with what I was missing. Elizabeth understood, and, lending her voice to my spirit, she insisted he go.

He was still muttering his objections when they left at the end of the visiting period, but he had agreed. I knew he'd go, if only for me.

I watched the clock all afternoon, though I tried to concentrate on the Houston Oilers football game on my radio. When six o'clock came, I knew Bill was at the party—for both of us. In my imagination, I pictured us driving up to the Houston Country Club. I saw Bill in his dark blue suit and me in my green silk dress. We would know all the people there, though there were some I hadn't seen in ages. I tried to picture each of the women and what she would be wearing.

I made myself concentrate on them, blotting out the doctor, nurses, and respiratory therapist who were congregated at my bedside. "Tracheotomy," they were saying to me, but I refused to listen. I felt a needle pierce my throat. Pain! Then numbness. Rough hands. I must escape. I shut them out with closed eyelids and my fantasy. I was at the party with Bill. We always enjoyed company functions. After all, Shell Oil Company had been so much a part of our finding one another.

When I graduated from SMU, I went to work in the accounting department at Shell. It was during the recession of 1958, but fortunately they were interested in the business half of my business/home economics degree. I'd taken that double major because I hadn't known what I wanted to do, and it seemed practical. At Shell, I was trained in all areas of the accounting department, and I found my niche in personnel and payroll. I was soon aware that the married people in accounting were trying to push the young singles together. And I was one of their targets.

The company was recruiting for the bowling leagues, and the people in my office encouraged me to get involved. Though I had taken bowling as a physical education course in college, I grew up in an era and in a community where a bowling alley was not considered the nicest place for a young lady to be seen. Now, however, in Houston, women's and mixed leagues were in full swing. Still, I was reluctant.

Finally, I signed up for the Friday night mixed league. I was uncomfortable at first, but the team members were very nice to me.

One Friday night we bowled a team that had this Bill Baier on it. He was a terrific bowler, rolling one strike after another. You could tell he was pretty proud of how he was doing. I was keeping score, and each time he bowled, he came to check whether I scored all his strikes properly. It perturbed me that he thought I didn't know how to add. After all, I was an accountant! It was obvious he was showing off, but he was nice looking, and I couldn't help noticing him.

The following day, I quietly looked in the company records to find out more about this great bowler.

Alarm! Whose? Voices.

"Turn that thing off! Get some suction here." The doctor's voice was demanding. Urgency surrounded me.

Please help, Bill. Bill!

I forced concentration on Bill Baier. I must get free of this madness, of all these people. They cannot harm me if I am not here. Bill and I . . . at Shell Oil Company. . . .

I commuted to work every day from Richmond, Texas, a small community some twenty-five miles southwest of Houston. One day as I drove to work, a car pulled out in front of me. I recognized *him*. That's how I discovered where he lived and the fact that he was in a car pool. Strangely, it happened again every morning thereafter. Just as I hit this one intersection, there came that little gray-and-white Ford carrying Bill Baier to work. The timing was uncanny. I could not help but become more aware of Bill Baier.

Eventually Bill got around to asking me out for lunch—to see if I was "worth" taking out to dinner, he later explained. That's when I learned for the first time what a practical man this was. He was twenty-eight years old and was no longer interested in dating just to go out and have a good time. He'd decided he was beyond all that foolishness.

One day, shortly after the lunch, Bill walked up to me at work and asked, "What would this one do if he would like to have a date with someone who lived way down in Richmond?"

And I answered, "One drives to Richmond and picks one up is

what one does." He smiled and nodded. I felt it wouldn't be too much longer before he called.

It was quiet now. They were all gone. Whatever they had had to do was finished. I wanted to stay awake and wait for Bill to come back from the party, but I could feel myself slipping away. The respirator hissed its pattern—zummm, tch . . . zumm, tch. . . . I tried to see what time it was, but the clock drifted off. And so did I.

When I woke up, Bill was standing beside my bed. How long had he been there? Our time together was too limited to waste any of it sleeping. As soon as I opened my eyes, he leaned over and kissed me tenderly. He was wearing his blue suit, just as I had imagined. Immediately he was swabbing out my mouth.

"They called me at the party and told me they were doing the trach. I'm sorry I wasn't here with you." Oh, Bill. I didn't want you here for that. You had to be at the party for both of us. "Was it painful?" he asked.

No. There was no way to tell him that only my thoughts of him, of us, fought off the fear and the pain.

"Everyone asked about you, wanted to know where you were. When I told them, they all sent their best wishes." Everyone. That's not good enough. I made him spell with me.

Who?

He began with the names. That was better. Familiar names. I had wondered who would be on the guest list.

"Oh, yes. Ann and Howard were there, and they were very upset to hear. . . ."

Ann and Howard. I felt an inner smile just thinking of them. We had such good times with them during our year in Holland, when we were all assigned to The Hague on the company exchange program. It's been so long since we've seen them. I must call Ann when I get out of the hospital.

". . . and Ann sent her love."

I was feeling tired now, very tired. And disappointed. I had really looked forward to this party; now it was over. Bill hadn't wanted to go alone, but he went for me, knowing I wanted to hear about it. And I did. But now I was too tired to listen any more. I love you, Bill, I whispered wordlessly as he kissed me good night and left.

Monday morning started off badly: I was assigned to Sandra. She seemed to mean well, but when something or someone distracted her, she'd scoot off, saying, "I'll be back in a few minutes, Sue."

On Sunday, Vickie, the best nurse I'd had since coming into intensive care, noticed on my chart that my bowels hadn't moved. "I'd better give you an enema," she said. "I hate to do it to you, but it's in your best interest." She was sincere, and I knew she was right. Later in the afternoon, the enema caused some minor happenings, but it never really took hold.

When Sandra came in on Monday morning, I tried to tell her what I needed. She just laughed. "Sue, you couldn't need a bedpan." Then something at the nurses' station caught her attention. "I'll be back in just a minute, Sue." And off she went.

Come back, come back! I could feel the impending rush, but I had no control. All of a sudden it was there. Terrible. All over the bed. I was horrified, humiliated. And angered because Sandra had betrayed me.

When she returned, her expression was one of amazement. "Oh, that *was* what you were trying to tell me."

Maybe now you will pay attention to me, I scolded her mentally. But that was no consolation. Through the cleanup she remained very kind and gentle, but I knew that she was perturbed. However, my thoughts of Sandra were short-lived, for now I realized I had lost control over all body functions. How could I possibly deal with this new humiliation? What more is there to lose? How far will this go? I fought for courage.

Bill had been so reassuring. He had tried to explain what he heard from the neurologist—that everything might go, but then it would return. I believed Bill. He was never one to say something unless it was so. I must believe. I didn't know what it would be like when everything shut down, but I did believe it would all come back. And the staff had told me about another patient with Guillain-Barré who had returned to a normal existence in three months. That was such a long time, but I could make three months. I believed and trusted. I was terrified, but I knew for certain that everything was going to come back again, even this control. I prayed it would come soon. I could endure just about anything, but not this. Please, not this.

Bill was waiting for Sandra to finish changing me. At least he hadn't seen what happened. He couldn't stay long. He had another meeting, so he had to leave in a few minutes. That was all right. I needed time to deal with this new degradation.

Thoughts of my father haunted me throughout this morning. What had gone through his mind during his lucid moments at the nursing home? Toward the end, he was bedridden, unable to move except to eat. I could see him lying there, and now it made me wonder. . . . I'd been so sure he was getting wonderful care. Still, I wondered whether some of these things happened to him, with Mother and me unaware and never able to help him.

Daddy had never lost his propriety, even as his senility worsened. The staff at the home said that most people who reach that point lose control over their thoughts. Though they may have been very nice people, they might give vent to some very unexpected words or gestures. The nurses said they had never seen such a gentleman in that state as my father. To the end, he was apologizing if he burped.

What had poor Daddy been through as he lost his bodily functions? I felt a new anguish for him—even as I felt it for myself.

Promptly at eleven-thirty, Bill returned. He looked so tired. How could he not be tired? So much to do. Each day he added new notations to his pocket journal.

He'd just been handed my first week's hospital bill and was studying it item by item. We were stunned by what this illness was costing. Every little thing was listed on the statement. We were both astounded by the charges for facial tissues, so Bill made a note to start bringing my brand from home. I liked them better than the hospital tissues, anyway. We would try to economize however we could.

Another note for Bill's book: batteries for the radio. They

lasted only two days, so Bill always had to remember to buy new ones. Soon, however, he bought a battery charger. Then he'd come in each day with fresh batteries in his pocket and take the used ones home to be recharged. I urgently needed the reality of that radio between his visits.

Each time we began to spell, the little diary came out, and Bill recorded my needs and my concerns. If those concerns required him to talk to a nurse or doctor, he did that, too.

And always I wanted to know about the girls. Had he talked to Katherine? Was Elizabeth going somewhere this evening? I'd known those things before and I still needed to know. I felt I *had* to remain involved with my family.

Never was there time enough to spell all the things I needed to say, to ask all the questions. But we had found a way to speed up the process. Now, before starting each word, I told him how many letters it had. When I indicated more than six or seven, he sputtered, "Can't you think of a shorter word?"

No! If I could, I would. The pressure of the fifteen-minute time limit created tension for both of us. There was so little time; none for me to say or ask anything beyond the barest essentials. Each time he came, I wanted to ask, "How are you, Bill? Are you getting enough rest? How are things at work?" But there was never enough time. And how I wanted to say, "I love you."

"December 9: Why Sue?"

—from Bill's diary

Bill was gone, and I wanted to rest, but I discovered that there was little of that to be found in a hospital.

In the early afternoon, a new person came to look at the dials on my respirator. A few seconds later, my very good friend Bess came in. I was so happy to see her that it never even occurred to me to worry about my appearance. After all, this was Bess. After a warm greeting, she pointed in the direction of the man at the dials. "Sue, I want you to meet someone. This is my friend Gary Stiller. We used to be neighbors." I was puzzled.

"Hello, Sue." After glancing at me briefly, he was again looking at Bess.

"Gary is in charge of the physical therapy department here, Sue," Bess explained. She was talking so fast that I could tell she was uncomfortable. "At one time he was also the head of respiratory therapy, so he knows about everything that's being done for you now. He'll be keeping an eye on you now, I'm sure."

Gary said he would be overseeing all of my physical therapy and also be very much involved in my case. He seemed interested and considerate. "Are you comfortable?"

I blinked once, but he didn't notice. But as with so many of the others here, he seemed uncomfortable addressing me, so he directed his questions to Bess. I was just an inanimate object lying between them. I stared steadily at him and fiercely blinked my answers. He did not notice. Each question was addressed to Bess. But she didn't know how to spell with me yet, so she could answer only with bits of information that Bill had given her.

Finally he gave up. "Well, I'd best be going."

To Bess he said, "Thanks for coming. I'll leave you two alone to visit. Just a few minutes, though."

And to me: "I'll be seeing you, Sue. If ever you need anything special, just ask for me."

It was so good to be alone with Bess, who was holding my hand and talking to me. I had the first news of her and our friends in a week. It seemed more like months. But a one-way conversation was awkward for her, and the few minutes were gone quickly.

Tears of frustration poured from my eyes when she left. How lucky I was to have a friend like Bess. Yet, now she could leave and her life went on as usual. But I was still imprisoned here in Bed Number Ten.

6

I closed my eyes, wanting to shut out the chaotic world surrounding me. Then I became aware of someone standing beside me. Another nurse? Another repositioning? More anxiety.

Finally, I opened my eyes, and there he stood—a man in a blue lab coat who had perhaps the broadest, warmest smile I'd ever seen. Even his large, dark-framed glasses could not dim the radiance beaming from his eyes.

"Hello, Sue. My name is Charles. I'm a physical therapist." He had taken my hand, as if to shake it, but instead held it gently in his large, comfortable hands. "I'm going to be working with you, starting tomorrow." He spoke directly to me, never looking away even for an instant. "We're just going to do a little range of motion with you. It's nothing to worry about."

Yes. I felt certain there was nothing to worry about. I knew instinctively that Charles would never deceive me.

"I'll be coming in twice a day, just working on your circulation. I am sure it will make you feel more comfortable."

Yes. I knew improving my circulation would definitely make me more comfortable.

"After you're a little better, we'll be taking you to the physical therapy department for regular work to rebuild your strength."

Yes. Yes! Charles was the first person here who spoke concretely of my getting better. And he was saying it directly to me, not talking to Bill or some other person on the other side of my bed!

Gently, he laid my hand back on the bed. "I'll see you tomorrow, Sue." The smile was still there, warm and sincere, as he waved good-bye. At least now there would be something different, something pleasant to anticipate.

As usual, I was watching the clock, waiting for Bill. My shoulder was sore. Why? I couldn't see my upper torso to look at what

54

was hurting. It was five-forty. Please come, Bill. And then he was there.

He'd been talking to a Dr. Langos, who told him they put in a "subclavian," a new term for both of us. Bill explained that it was an intravenous feeding tube that was inserted in my shoulder area.

Bill was studying my right shoulder. "It will be used instead of the IV that was in your arm." A couple of stitches held the subclavian in place, he told me. Sadly, I realized that meant it was intended to stay there for some time.

I couldn't remember anything about the procedure, except people hovering over me. I'd fought them out of my consciousness. The doctor told Bill they used a local anesthetic and did it right there in my bed. It only took a few minutes, he said.

I'd also been given a nasogastric tube, an NG tube for short. I remembered that procedure. A nurse, Phil, had been instructed to insert the tube, which had to go up my nose, down my throat, and straight into my stomach. He'd tried and tried, but apparently he couldn't get it past a small growth in my nostril. I felt as if I were a rag doll, being put into a horrible angle to try to make it work. He was a tall, slender man who was rough when he tried to do anything. He'd been that way when he'd put the IV in my arm several days earlier. But now he seemed to be thinking, "I'm going to get this down you or else." An absolute nightmare.

Phil never spoke to me, even to tell me what he was trying to do or that he was sorry it was so difficult for me. I don't think he realized I was conscious. Finally he gave up and a doctor came back to do it. In spite of the agony and fear, I'd felt surges of anger as they worked on me. And I kept thinking of Bruce's warning that first night: "Get used to that. You're going to have a lot of that while you're here."

"The doctors are concerned because you're losing weight so drastically," Bill said. "They have to provide you with more food." From now on, I would be fed supplements through the NG tube, plus regular IVs through the subclavian. They were forcing nourishment down me as fast as possible.

How nice! A tube for everything. I counted them: these two, the respirator, the Foley catheter, and four sensors that "plugged" me into the nursing station monitors. Those had been hooked up as a routine procedure when I first came into intensive care, to check my heart and respiration. What else was I to be wired to before this was over?

Bill reported that he'd had a long phone conversation with Dr. Lohmann, who told him I was doing very well. What on earth could he have meant by "doing very well"?

"He assured me that you're being stabilized and your condition is not critical. He said you're in good hands here." All these tubes and cords to keep me alive, and I'm not critical. And "in good hands," indeed. Whose? When my bed was tilted, with the head elevated, I could see the staff go from one patient to the next—often without ever washing those "good hands."

Dr. Lohmann also told Bill they were taking me off cortisone. In some cases it lightens the symptoms of Guillain-Barré somewhat, he had said, but there was no indication it was helping me. However, my infection was responding to the antibiotics. At least there was one reason to be thankful.

Poor Bill had been through another hectic day, but now he relaxed for a few minutes and reported on his accomplishments. He never mentioned work, just what he'd managed to do for me. Last night after leaving the hospital, he finished addressing the Christmas cards to our friends in Holland. These were people we knew so well, and I always enjoyed writing letters to go with the cards. Writing those letters seemed to mark the beginning of the holiday season for me. But this year I could only lie here and think about those friends. Another sadness.

Just before I got sick, we had purchased a new washing machine. Now Bill told me it was being delivered tomorrow. Mother would go to our house and wait for the truck. He had also talked to my friend Liz about taking a few house plants, especially the orchids. They had belonged to Liz's mother, a special friend. She and I had shared an interest in them, and after her death, Liz gave me her orchids. Keeping them alive was important to me. Now Liz would keep them at her house while I was in the hospital. Bill also asked Liz's advice about the rest of our plants. She had cared for them the year we were in Holland and knew our jungle nearly as well as I did.

My bromeliads, he informed me, were also being well cared for. My collection, made up of seven lovely varieties, had been started by a friend. B.G., as everyone knew her, had hundreds of plants, two greenhouses full of them. She knew all of her bromeliads by their botanical names. First she had given me one of them. Then, after I sent her a picture of the foot-and-a-half-long flower spike—to prove I'd been successful—she gave me another, and then another, until I had seven. She'd heard I was in the hospital for a long stay, so yesterday she stopped by to pick them up. What a relief for Bill! Seven fewer plants to care for.

Tonight, however, we had another, more serious concern to deal with, and Bill finally got to it. He and Mother had talked about the girls' party, and she was very much against their having it. She did not think the party was appropriate when I was in the hospital. So Bill would have to tell Elizabeth that Nana would not come to the party, or have anything to do with the preparations. This was incomprehensible to me! Life did have to go on, just as I had expected things to go on with my Bridge Club. If only I could talk with her myself. Mother has always been so good with party planning and table decorations. I was sure she'd help Elizabeth—and Katherine after she got home from school. It would give them something to share now, when they all needed one another. I was so disappointed—and bewildered. But there was nothing to be done about that now. Bill would not intrude on her decision, and I could not. He'd just have to tell Elizabeth she was on her own.

For a change, I had some good news tonight—my starting physical therapy. But how could I tell Bill in the little time we had? I began spelling. *Charles.*

He was puzzled. A nurse walked past my cubicle, and Bill stopped her to ask, "Who is Charles?"

She smiled at me and told Bill, "That's one of our physical therapists. I think he's going to start Sue on range of motion tomorrow. He's excellent."

"Is that what you were trying to tell me, Sue? Was he here to see you?"

Yes.

"Are you concerned about what he'll be doing?"

No.

"Well, you must have liked him."

Yes.

"Hmmm." Bill pulled out his diary and slowly, with exagger-ated syllables, articulated the words he was writing. "En-ter Char-les." This was the first time I'd been aware of any humor since I arrived in ICU. It felt good.

Our pastor from St. Philip, Sam Lanham, stopped by—a pleasant surprise. He did not always make such calls because our congregation had a special minister assigned to hospital visitation. I was concerned; my condition must really be serious for Sam to come. Perhaps he was here because he and Bill were associates through their church activities. Yes, that must be the reason. After all, Bill said I was not critical.

Sam had a special way with words, and his thoughts and prayers were just what we both needed.

Finally, Bill had to leave. Friends from church were meeting him here at the hospital to give him a casserole for dinner. I was so pleased, and Bill was relishing a meal he and Elizabeth didn't have to cook. Neither of us could have guessed that this was only the start of a great outpouring of such kindness. In the months ahead, our friends and neighbors and the wonderful people of St. Philip would see to that.

The evening looked long and bleak, as it always did after Bill left. So many hours of emptiness. So many hours of terror at being all alone. Whenever a nurse or respiratory therapist left me, I was seized with horrible fear, knowing that I could not move or call for help, no matter what was happening to me. I watched the staff congregate in the nursing station—just a few feet away, yet so removed. They all seemed to be socializing. I wondered if anyone realized that I was frightened, lonely, and bored. Every now and then, when they remembered or it was convenient, they came out and did what had to be done—turned me, or checked an IV or the respirator, or forced a packet of feeding solution down my NG tube. There was not necessarily any schedule, and most of them were so impersonal.

That's not fair, Sue, I scolded myself. They can't be in here all the time with me. They'd go crazy spending all their hours with someone who can't even talk. And they have other patients to look after. They are watching the monitors. They know I'm all right. And I will be all right. I will. Dr. Lohmann says I am not critical. I'm stabilized. But I can't help it. I am so afraid to be alone.

Bill had turned on the radio as he left. At least there were voices to keep me company for the night. I concentrated on the six o'clock news. Traffic was snarled from a cloudburst on the west side of town. I hope Bill and Elizabeth made it home safely. Let me think. What meeting did she have today after school . . . ?

What a wonderful surprise when Jo came into view. I was so glad to see her again that I no longer felt embarrassed about how I looked. I *hadn't* frightened her away the first time she came!

"How good to see you," she said. She couldn't imagine how good it was for me to see her tonight! Her voice was music. She said that she had talked to Bill at church Sunday and asked if I knew the whole congregation was praying for me. I blinked once, and she seemed to understand instinctively that I was saying *yes*. "You signaled me with your eyes, didn't you?"

Yes.

"Wonderful. And what is your *no* response?" I blinked twice. "Well, then," she went on, "we can talk now. Are you in pain?"

No. That wasn't exactly true, but I couldn't possibly explain to her that a wrinkle in the sheet was causing my hip much discomfort. She talked of her children and mine, her husband's business travel, friends from church—just everyday things. How wonderful to share just a few simple details of a friend's life.

"December 10: Hospital switchboard says Sue 'still critical'! "
—from Bill's diary

I watched the morning shift making rounds. Nothing of significance was reported on Sue Baier. "Sue's stable." It was as if they were saying, "You don't really need to worry about Sue any more. She's stable." Here I was, unable to move, unable to breathe, and the message seemed to be, don't worry about Sue. After all, we've got a heart attack over here, and so-and-so had an operation, but Sue's fine. I wanted to shout: Hey, wait a minute. You're not in intensive care if you're OK.

They said I had a restful night. In frustration I thought about the previous night. I'd been force-fed a dietary supplement at two o'clock. After feeding me, my night nurse—she was new to me—rolled me over, and the metal clamp from my NG tube was caught under my shoulder. It was two hours before she came back to reposition me and ended the agony. I'm not sure she noticed it even then. She just accidentally rolled me off of it. And now she was reporting that I had slept well!

I studied the faces of the morning group and wondered if there was someone who would try to communicate with me. That was always my first waking, anxious thought.

Now they were gone, and I was left to stare at the clock, ticking off the hour until Bill's arrival. In minutes, however, a friendly face appeared at the foot of the bed. Charles. He was carrying a steaming cup of coffee as he stood there smiling at me.

"I just stopped by to see how you are doing and to check whether you are going to be ready for me today." He nodded his head in the direction of the nurses' station. "They say you're doing fine. Are they right?"

Two blinks. But he didn't need the sign; he could read the expression in my eyes.

"That's what I thought. They always say everyone is fine." Once again I felt like smiling—if only I could. He read my bemusement, and his smile acknowledged it, before becoming a little more serious.

"Are you going to be ready for some range of motion this morning?"

Yes. Yes, yes, yes.

Again the smile. "Well, that was emphatic. I'll see you after your bath." I could hardly wait.

Bill came in, reporting that the casserole had been delicious. I'd known it would be a great treat. As he started to tell me about Elizabeth's plans for the day, the man Bess had brought in yesterday walked up to the foot of my bed and introduced himself to Bill. Gary Stiller. Yes, that was his name. He immediately began talking about tennis shoes. *Tennis shoes!* Bill's expression displayed the surprise I felt.

"What she needs are some high-topped tennis shoes, something stiff and heavy to keep her feet firm and upright." He was actually serious about this. And *high-topped* tennis shoes at that. "Without them, she'll get foot-drop."

Bill was giving him full attention while I lay there thinking that they were out of their minds. Here I was, burning up with heat, and even though my feet often felt cool to the touch, they had been sweating terribly. I cringed at the thought. Most of the time my hospital baths were no more than a wipe with a wet washcloth. They never think to wash my feet! People were already being a little careless about handling me. Those tennis shoes would be heavy and clumsy every time they turned me. But worst of all, I could just picture myself lying in that bed, tubes coming from everywhere—six feet tall, covered only with a skimpy little hospital gown, and wearing *high-topped tennis shoes!*

"When all the muscular control is gone, the foot falls forward," Gary was explaining. "If we don't brace it, her foot will get to the point that we can't get it back at an angle again." I didn't want foot-drop, but there had to be something other than those ridiculous tennis shoes. Surely there was another way.

Gary was gone, and Bill still stood there very seriously considering his newest challenge. I wanted him to laugh and tell me how silly this was. But he took out his pocket diary and made a note—to look for the tennis shoes, of course.

I signaled. *No, no, no.* But Bill was too preoccupied to notice. He kissed me and took off for his office—and his quest for high-topped tennis shoes!

After Bill left, I tried to forget such nonsense. I was ready to get on with my bath before Charles came to begin my therapy.

But *bath* was hardly the word for what I would get today. Immediately I sensed friction between the nursing staff and the physical therapy department.

"We'll have to make this short today, Sue," Linda said. "We're a little behind, and Charles will be here soon to work with you. You know how that goes." I didn't know—not yet. But I would learn that, too. The barely damp washcloth skimmed over my exposed skin. "There, that should hold you for now." Couldn't she see the perspiration that poured off me or the oil that must have made my skin shine? Imagine *tennis shoes*! What I wouldn't give for a long, warm shower, with soap and shampoo.

Linda neatly pulled the sheet and blanket up over my shoulders and gave me a professional pat. "There."

No. Please, not the covers. Desperately I tried to signal her, but she disappeared with the towel and one barely damp washcloth.

Within minutes, Charles came. Already my face was covered with moisture. "You look terribly warm, Sue. Why don't I just take these covers off?"

Yes. Oh, thank you!

"Now, just relax. I'm not going to do anything to hurt you." Slowly, gently, he began to work my hands, my fingers, my arms, massaging them and moving them around. Then he did the same with my feet, toes, and legs. Everything was limp, but I could feel the muscles moving and responding to his steady kneading. Even as he studied the appendage he was working on, he looked frequently at my eyes, watching for any hint of discomfort. There was none. It just felt good to know my blood was still circulating. As he worked, he chatted about the weather, his department, the news of the day. His personal commentary was much better than radio headlines.

Before leaving, Charles asked if I wanted to be covered.

No. I felt comfortable and relaxed for the moment, and I was very grateful he thought to ask.

"Then I'll see you this afternoon." I seldom had the same nurse two days in a row. Was there really going to be one person in this hospital that I could count on day after day?

Just after Bill's noon visit, San Williams, our minister of pastoral care, arrived. He was the person assigned to hospital visitation. San was a tall, lean, clean-cut young man. The wisdom in his eyes belied his age.

He spoke directly and sincerely. "You know, it must really be hard to just lie there and look around." He understood! He zeroed in on my fears, on my feelings of desperate loneliness. He had brought me a book of psalms from the Bible.

"I'll leave this here. Then we can read from it whenever you'd like."

Yes. His smile told me he read my response.

"Sue, may I read a psalm now?"

Again, *Yes.*

Slowly, he opened the book and thumbed through to the Forty-sixth Psalm. His soothing voice made the words come alive.

God is our refuge and strength, a very present help in trouble.
Therefore will not we fear, though the earth be removed, and though the mountains be carried into the midst of the sea;
Though the waters thereof roar and be troubled, though the mountains shake with the swelling thereof.
There is a river, the streams whereof shall make glad the city of God, the holy place of the tabernacles of the most High.
God is in the midst of her; she shall not be moved: God shall help her, and that right early. . . .

7

The curtain at my right was losing some of its sterile plainness. Bright, cheerful greeting cards sprouted into view when I was turned to my side. Get-well cards had begun arriving almost immediately—some at the hospital, others at home.

The first three arrived at home on the same day, and Bill brought them in the next morning. After reading each one to me and holding them so I could see them, he began to put the three envelopes back into his coat pocket. Carol saw him and said, "You're not going to take them back home, are you?" Before a startled Bill Baier could respond to this earnest question, she continued: "Why don't we just hang them on the curtain for Sue to enjoy?"

Again not waiting for an answer, she hurried off to the nurses' station to get masking tape. While Bill and I watched, Carol attached the cards to the curtain, directly in my line of vision. I loved it! Later in the morning, when I was lying on my back, watching the clock, the perky flowers on Elaine's card caught my attention. I could just see them with my peripheral vision, and they provided a beautiful touch of the outside world.

Soon the first Snoopy card arrived, and inside was the signature, "George," and the paw print of his dachshund, Hure. George was an old friend of Bill's from early in their careers when they worked in West Texas. They have remained very good friends over the years. Still a bachelor, George now works for a government office in the District of Columbia. He's been like an uncle to the girls, always sending them interesting gifts from his travels around the world. His gifts arrive without fanfare—no birthday, no special occasion. They just arrive.

The first week there were three Snoopy cards, all from George and Hure. The shape is so easily recognizable that soon I could spot the long, narrow envelope sticking out from the stack in

Bill's hand. I'd smile to myself, knowing there was another card from George with Hure's paw print.

In the weeks to come, as the curtain was being covered with cards, each new addition became a link with the thoughtful person who sent it. The brightness of the cards and the warmth of the messages brought me much cheer.

While Hure's paw print amused me, it also reminded me of our cat, Tiffany. She was still quite young, and I was concerned about her. She was accustomed to being in the house whenever I was home. But now, with me gone, she had to be shut outside all day. Bill said she always cried when he got home at night and was so happy to see him. Poor Tiffany. Along with worrying about everyone else, I worried about her.

But that was nothing new. We always seemed to have a cat that needed worrying about. One year, we all worried through the birth of a litter that Katherine believed was her birthday present.

I had been relaxing in the family room after getting the girls to bed. It was the night before Katherine's birthday, so I was doing a last-minute checklist on birthday party arrangements. Somehow the cat had slipped upstairs. Bill saw her on Katherine's bed when he went up for his shower, but he decided to leave her until he finished. Before long, Katherine's sleepy little head came through the door to the family room and she said, "Mother, I think I heard a kitten cry in my bed." Sure enough, there lay mama cat, purring happily as she cleaned off her new baby. Of course, Elizabeth woke up and came running in, too.

I had grown up with cats, but this was all new to Bill and the girls. So we had prepared ahead by reading and talking about cats and kittens. We knew the new mother and babies should not be moved far from the place of the first delivery, so Bill got the box we'd prepared for the new family and placed it at the foot of Katherine's bed, where we all settled in to watch the rest of the births.

When the third kitten arrived, the mother pushed it aside and wouldn't clean it. Bill had read that a cat senses when there is something wrong with an offspring, and she won't try to help it at all. We got a doll's bottle and made a formula of honey and milk, but the poor little thing never did drink.

We stayed up all through the birthing—a night for us to share. Of course, the next day we all struggled sleepily through the birthday party, but for a long time we talked about that special night.

At home now, Bill and Elizabeth were getting into some interesting situations. She needed money for the usual minor purchases—small clothing items, school supplies. This was the first time Bill had to concern himself with the girls' daily expenses. I could only smile ruefully to myself. Welcome to another facet of family life, Bill Baier!

Katherine was having exams at Vanderbilt. Bill still hadn't told her exactly how ill I was; she didn't need that concern during her first-semester exams. It was unusual for us to conceal anything serious from our daughters, but this time it had to be. Katherine would be home soon enough, and then he could tell her the truth. At least by that time the stress of exams would be over.

Back on my first day in ICU, Margie Hood had stopped by to see me. I'd been very surprised when she walked in wearing a volunteer's uniform. I hadn't known she volunteered at Gulfland Hospital. On that day, she was just going off duty, but she promised to visit me regularly.

Margie was a good friend from our exchange year in The Hague. Both our husbands had been assigned to Holland for the same year. I'd known Archie Hood in the days when I was passing out pay envelopes at Shell. Some of the men would tease me because I was the new, young graduate, but Archie was a quiet, sweet person who always put me at ease. So when I learned we were going to The Hague along with Archie and his wife, that was an added bonus.

Bill had been sent to the Netherlands to address a conference two years before the exchange. We'd made very elaborate plans for me to go along on that trip because we were sure that would be our only chance to go to Holland together. We'd had a beautiful week, and I'd fallen in love with The Hague.

One lovely evening, as we walked back to the hotel after dinner, I said to Bill, "Wouldn't it be wonderful to come back and live here?"

"Sorry. I'm in the wrong part of the company for that ever to happen."

Then one afternoon two years later, Bill called from work. "Are you sitting down?"

"Yes." I was by the time I said it.

"We're being sent to The Hague for a year!"

The preparations were chaotic. Bill and I had to find someone to live in our house while we were gone, decide which things would go with us and which would go into storage, and get books for the girls' studies. But it was all worth it when we finally landed in The Hague. And visiting with Margie and Archie for the first time, I found he was as special as I'd remembered him, and Margie was just as nice.

Their children were grown and had remained in the United States, so in Holland we became one family. The six of us often traveled together for weekends. And of course we celebrated holidays with Margie and Archie, our extended family.

We kept in touch after returning to Houston, but Margie's volunteer work never came up in conversation. Now, I discovered that not only was she a volunteer, but she was currently president of the volunteers' organization. Wednesday was her regular day at the hospital; today, a week after her first visit, she was back—and so welcome.

Bill and Mother were obviously very happy to see Margie, too, a familiar face in this sea of strangers. Though volunteers did not work in ICU, she offered to help Bill with anything he might need.

It was not long before Bill did need Margie's help—to find a shampoo for me. I don't know how many days passed without anyone realizing my hair needed washing. I knew greasy hair was not a life-threatening situation, which is what intensive care is designed to accommodate, but I was miserable. I've always thought greasy blond hair was particularly unsightly.

One evening Luana, an Indonesian nurse, who was not my nurse that night, walked over and said, "Your hair needs washing. Do you know that?"

Hooray! Somebody has noticed! *Yes!*

"Is it all right with you if I call your husband and have him bring you some shampoo?"

Yes. Oh, thank you, Luana.

Her call, however, sent Bill into a tailspin. He had to start looking for an instant shampoo, knowing they would not be able to rinse my hair properly. He'd heard about the usual dry shampoos, but those powders, he felt, would just coat my oily hair. So he contacted Margie, who found exactly the right shampoo in the hospital gift shop—a liquid that could be used with or without water.

Several days passed before someone got around to doing my hair. It was a Sunday. Bill was at church and there would be no therapy for me, and this day there were no new critical patients in ICU. Harriet and Bonnie came to my bedside with the news: today I was getting a shampoo! Both had already endeared themselves to me. Harriet was the first person in the unit to speak kindly to me. And Bonnie's special introduction had occurred a couple of days ago, when she came to me before Bill arrived and washed my face. "Let's make you look nice for Bill," she said. And for once I did feel just a little better.

Now she and Harriet had the bottle of shampoo. "I don't know how we're going to do this," said Harriet, "but don't worry. We'll figure out something." How could I worry, listening to the two of them giggling?

"Bill says she has sensitive skin," Bonnie commented. "Even though the bottle says the stuff doesn't need to be rinsed out of her hair, I think we'd better not take a chance." I wanted to tell them that it wasn't sensitive in the way they thought. I was afraid they'd get discouraged and give up. While I tried to decide which words to spell, Harriet had an idea.

"A fracture pan!" she announced. "It'll be perfect." She dashed off to find one, and when she returned, I laughed silently with them.

"It *is* perfect," Bonnie proclaimed. And I had to agree. It was a plastic bedpan that is used for hip-surgery patients—similar to a regular bedpan but narrower, with a larger opening in the front. Using a pillow and towels, they propped up my head and it fit perfectly into the opening. They were like children with a doll, arranging me playfully but with care. How they laughed. I loved the sound and even being a silent part of it.

Other nurses passed by and joined the laughter. "Good grief! Y'all found a new use for the fracture pan," one said.

The only water in the cubicle was a little sink back in the corner, but no one ever seemed to be able to get warm water from it. So Bonnie went to get a pitcher of warm water, and the shampoo began. It was the nicest thing that had happened to me since I'd been there. The water felt heavenly. Their fingers massaged my scalp. This was real luxury. After the first rinse, they decided to do a second wash. Hooray! They understood how wonderful it felt. If only I could have smiled for them.

After the washing, Harriet said, "She's going to catch cold if we don't get that hair dry." Again there was laughter as they tried to hold my limp head and fluff the hair dry. Their hands felt so good! It was a glorious morning.

I'd been having some discomfort with my back, but I seldom let them give me anything for the pain because I didn't want any extra medication. But now Bonnie gave me a hypo to relax. With clean hair and a hypo, I was positioned comfortably on my side and I got my first good sleep since coming to the hospital. When I awoke, feeling clean and rested, I came alive, certain that things were going to get better.

The next morning, two new postoperative patients arrived in intensive care, and my assigned nurse announced she was overloaded. So it was back to the swish of a damp washcloth as my bath for the day.

Every once in a while, however, I got lucky again. Often that was when Vickie would be assigned to me for the day. Vickie was a superb nurse. I recognized that the first time she worked with me. She said she'd trained under Dr. Denton Cooley, the famous Houston heart surgeon. It was obvious she was experienced in intensive care nursing. Perhaps this is why she was assigned to me so seldom—her experience was needed with critically ill patients.

Vickie was a vibrant, outgoing person. As she washed me—with warm water and soap, real suds!—she laughed and talked to everyone in the unit. She brought life into my barren cubicle. When she talked with me, she actually communicated, telling me about her husband, who was in chiropractic school, and funny tales about her life at home. During a bath, she changed the water in the pan several times to keep it warm and fresh. Once when she was nearly finished, she looked at me with a mischievous grin and said, "Oh, it's no fun to lie here and not be able to get into the water." Then she put my feet into the pan, allowing me to enjoy the bath water. She actually recognized that I could *feel*! Such a rare pleasure.

And another wonder occurred with Vickie. She brushed my teeth! She looked at my mouth and said, "I don't know how we're going to do this, but there has to be a way. Your mouth must feel terribly uncomfortable."

Yes! It really did.

Since I had no muscle control, my mouth was stiff, and she could barely keep it open. Other nurses had mentioned my teeth, but they were afraid I might choke on the water. But Vickie was doing it! She had to suction out the water she used, as a dentist would. One little trickle going down the windpipe could create real problems. But having my teeth brushed was worth the risk. Vickie was one nurse who thoroughly understood long-term patient care.

The problem was becoming clearer to me. Intensive care was not a place for long-term patients. The staff was trained for the normal, specialized, life-support care of the critically ill. They were neither equipped nor prepared to handle a long-term, totally helpless patient. A wipe for a bath was acceptable for a day or two with a patient too sick to know or care. But regular baths, shampooing, and toothbrushing were not part of the routine of this department. Fortunately, to some of them these everyday procedures represented a challenge readily accepted—when time permitted.

Vickie never shied from the challenge. One time she had just turned me when she stopped to examine my bed. "Sue, you don't have an air mattress. I can't believe no one has thought of it. You really need one."

I had no idea what she was referring to. I did have one of the foam-rubber pads called an egg carton, because of the contours of the top surface. After the first few days, it provided very little protection to my spindly body. Indeed, I was being turned so often because everyone was greatly concerned about the possibility of my getting bedsores.

Off Vickie went to find an air mattress, but there wasn't one in the supply department. Undaunted, she searched the storage areas of the ICU and finally found one that had been used. "It's not brand new, Sue," she said, "but we'll fix that. Believe me, you won't mind a bit." She spread it out on the floor next to my bed, got down on her hands and knees, and started scrubbing—much to everyone's amazement. When any of the staff commented, Vickie said, "Sue needs one of these, so we're going to fix up this one." And she continued scrubbing. After she was satisfied that it was clean, Vickie took on the next hazard—getting it under me. She called to Marie for help. Marie usually worked the eleven-to-seven shift, but today it was her misfortune to be on in the morning. She was more than willing to help.

I am sure neither of them realized how difficult the job would be. They couldn't take me out of bed, because I was hooked up with the trach, subclavian, ICU monitors, and the catheter, so the mattress had to be inserted under the egg-carton pad *and* the sheet *and* me.

They lifted me by the sheet and I rolled helplessly from one side to the other. "Hang in there, Sue," Marie said again and again. "We'll be through in a few minutes." As they lifted the sheet and tried to hold onto the foam-rubber pad, they shoved in the air mattress a few inches at a time. I was being rolled around wildly, but there was nothing else they could do.

It was terrifying. My head was going in all directions, with saliva running out all over. Other staff told Vickie and Marie they were crazy as they struggled with me, but they never gave up. "Hang on, Sue, just a little longer," Vickie assured. Again my limp body was jostled from side to side.

I did hang on, convinced from what Vickie had said that this mattress would be well worth the struggle. And mentally I celebrated with the two of them when they finally finished— especially after they turned on the compressor that would keep it inflated. The air moved my body up and down in something like a breathing pattern. Fantastic! It shifted the pressure from one area to another, relieving some of the soreness. In spite of the frightening moments, I was very grateful to them both.

Later in the day, a janitor came in to mop the floor and accidentally unplugged the compressor. I lay there for two hours until I could signal a nurse who was turning me, and she reconnected the machine. This would happen often. But when the mattress was working, it helped tremendously.

Christmas was less than two weeks away and it was on my mind all the time. I was able to accept the fact that this was where I would spend my Christmas, but I was determined that Bill, the girls, and my mother were going to have a Christmas, regardless. I plagued Bill with things to do. His visits were sometimes a little longer now. The staff seemed to realize I was more relaxed when he was there, so his visits were a relief for them, too. After I told Bill about a wrinkle in the sheet, or a nurse who couldn't understand me, I began with Christmas instructions.

After Bill mailed the cards to the Netherlands, he informed me, "I am not going to go through your whole Christmas card list." I protested. I had already purchased the cards. Finally he compromised. As cards arrived, Bill prepared one in return and wrote a brief note about where I was. Oh, I wished I could write my own cards, but I was thankful the cards were being sent.

The staff began decorating the ICU for Christmas. With all her exuberance, Vickie climbed up and down a ladder, hanging garlands around the top of the nursing station. Bless them all. I knew they were trying to bring a touch of holiday cheer into the lives of the patients. But, while I appreciated their efforts, it was disheartening. I'd heard that Christmas is for many people the most depressing time of year, and I had never comprehended that before.

As the decorating continued, I kept thinking back to the first Christmas Daddy spent in the nursing home. Like him, most of the patients in the home appeared senile. When they were singing Christmas carols and eating Christmas cookies, he seemed oblivious. Now I couldn't help but wonder what was going through Daddy's mind that Christmas. Had he known it was Christmas and been unable to tell us?

Tears flowed down my cheeks. I longed to be home, decorating my house, preparing for my family's Christmas. A radio commercial rang out, "I'll be home for Christmas. . . ." But I won't. I can't.

8

Bill started his vacation on December 15. We always tried to save part of his vacation for the holidays when the girls were out of school, and this year he'd saved two weeks for when Katherine came home from school. Now that time had come.

Bill was meeting Katherine's plane. I couldn't wait to see her. It seemed an eternity since she was home—since we *both* were home for Thanksgiving weekend. That Saturday she and I had gone shopping and out to lunch, alone together with time to talk. She told me all the things a mother waits so long to hear—about our relationship and what it meant to her. I was so touched. As she left for Nashville the next afternoon, I counted the days until she would be back, planning how our new relationship could just start up again where we left off.

Finally she was at my bedside, almost frozen in place, trying not to show her shock and disbelief. I knew how I looked. I saw in the faces of so many visitors the reflection of my own emaciated appearance. How difficult this must be for her. Driving from the airport, Bill surely tried to prepare her for this moment, but who could prepare anyone for this—the gauntness, the tubes and machinery. There is no way to condition someone for a reality such as this.

Bill looked drained. Obviously it had not been an easy trip for either of them. Had it been the right decision to delay telling her everything? How I wanted to hold this child, my firstborn, in my arms. I wanted desperately to spare her this shock and horror. Elizabeth had watched me slip away; she'd been able to adjust gradually to my illness. But for Katherine, the overwhelming reality was hitting her all at once.

Trouper that she was, after barely a moment's pause, she began on the news I was so anxious to hear. "I think I passed all my exams." Finally she was smiling, that impish grin that said she was feigning modesty. Katherine had won a number of scholastic awards before graduating from high school; I knew she would do well in college. But still I wanted to know about it all from her. It was good to hear about her classes, new friends, campus life. There were no awkward silences. Bill taught her how to spell with me, and she "listened" and answered with animation. I was enormously relieved at how well she was handling the shock. Only months later could Mother tell me that after Katherine left the hospital, she broke down and sobbed, "That can't be my mother!"

The hospital staff was increasingly preoccupied with Christmas. Most of them had families, and, as with other working people, their minds were on decorating homes or apartments, shopping, and holiday meal preparations—all the rushing-around that had to be done after they left work.

"Have to go shopping tonight," Elaine said almost every day. She made it sound like drudgery. I wished I could go shopping. I especially loved Christmas shopping. But then I didn't have to go to work eight hours a day and try to squeeze in my shopping during the crowded evening hours. Getting ready for Christmas *was* my job, normally, this time of year, and I thoroughly enjoyed it. Perhaps that is why I never thought about going back to work after Katherine and Elizabeth were born. When I had my family, I had found the only career I ever wanted, and I was fortunate to have been able to stay home all those years.

As I listened to all the talk of Christmas preparations, I was faced with a frightening reality. In spite of all my frustrations with many of the staff, I had met some excellent nurses and therapists. But now, just as we were establishing rapport, they were talking about taking vacations over the holidays. I was doomed to facing strangers once again, just when I had started to relax with a few familiar people, to look forward to a friendly smile or a kind gesture—such as when Donna stopped in late at night to wash my face, comb my hair, and freshen my mouth with a lemon swab. Or the extra moment she took early in the morning to turn on my radio before going off duty. The break between the night shift's last services and Bill's arrival was particularly desolate. Everyone was busy doing paperwork, making rounds, and reassembling for the new day, and I always felt so isolated. It helped to listen to the weather and traffic reports, the overnight news, and the announcer's light chatter. I was so thankful when Donna was my nurse, and now, when I'd just begun to look forward to her special kindnesses, she was talking about going to California for two weeks over the holidays.

Three respiratory therapists had become mainstays of my existence in ICU. Others who were good came and went. But these three I could rely on. Peter was on days. He and Charles, the physical therapist, were housemates, and that seemed to draw Peter more closely into what I was feeling and needing. James, who worked the second shift, was a close friend of both men, and, like Charles and Peter, he began immediately to communicate with me.

My third respiratory therapist was Kay. The first time I saw her, she was working a day shift. Immediately I liked the sound of her—jovial and full of fun. She explained to Bill all the procedures for cleaning and adjusting the respirator, and showed him how the water level must be watched. I was very attentive also. I'd never noticed anyone checking that water level, but I surely would keep track of it from now on. I was beginning to feel that my survival in ICU might well depend on my knowing everything about my care.

When Kay began working weeknights regularly, I felt a little measure of security. At least during the week, there was usually one person on each shift who came to me at regular intervals, checked the respirator, and suctioned me, and who cared enough to spell with me and ask if I was all right.

But now all three therapists were talking about Christmas holidays and time off. Panic gripped me. How would I manage to communicate without them?

My mind raced for a solution. Facing the prospect of so many new substitutes over the holidays, I had to find some way to let them know what I needed. When Katherine returned the next day with Bill, I had an idea.

Need chart, I spelled.

"What kind of chart?" they asked simultaneously.

Questions.

They looked at each other and then back to me. Suddenly the idea clicked with Bill.

"You want a chart with questions so the staff can find out what you need." It was half question and half answer.

Yes!

They agreed it might work. Already Katherine saw in my eyes how desperate I was to communicate. One by one I indicated the questions we needed to incorporate. Hot? Cold? Radio on? Radio off? They all had to be *yes* and *no* answers. Back hurt? Turn? Eye drops? (From all the blinking, my eyes were getting terribly dry, so Dr. Lohmann prescribed eye drops for use whenever I needed them. Getting someone to put them in was another matter.)

Bill and Katherine left in pursuit of the new challenge, and the next day they returned with my chart. It was simple and straightforward—and I hoped it would work. They hung it on the wall behind my bed, under the number ten.

For a few staff members the system worked, but, sadly, many totally ignored it. Even some who looked at it seemed puzzled. They just shrugged their shoulders, and their impatient expressions said, I'm not going to bother with that nonsense. For them I was still a silent object without awareness or personal needs.

I pleaded with Bill for private nurses, but Dr. Lohmann informed Bill that this was not permitted in ICU. Besides, the head nurse had assured him I was getting excellent care. It was clear to me I had to get out of this unit, but that was impossible as long as I needed the respirator. I was crumbling under defeat.

Ignored. Repeatedly I tried to tell Bill how frightened and frustrated I was.

This morning it happened again. My nurse refused to acknowledge any need to communicate and dumped me into a heap after what was supposed to be my bath. How I wished for

Bonnie again. She'd been so understanding yesterday, giving me a good bath, spelling with me, trying to be attentive.

Now my back was sagging and my neck was twisted. I looked for someone to help me. Bonnie walked past on her way to the bed next to me. Surely she would get me straightened out. Frantically I blinked my eyes, trying to get her attention. She did not see me. Soon, en route to the nurses' station, she stopped directly in front of my bed to respond to someone's question. Again I tried to signal her, but she never looked at me. It was as though my bed were unoccupied. All through the shift I watched her going back and forth, this nurse who had been so empathetic yesterday. Today I was not her patient, and I was invisible. I felt betrayed, bewildered by her seeming rejection.

When I spelled this frustration to Bill, he tried to understand, and it obviously saddened him. There was nothing he could do but reassure me that I was safe and would be taken care of. After all, Dr. Lohmann told him I was in good hands. Perhaps they all thought I was too sick to know what was happening or what I was saying.

Every day I asked Bill to call the doctor and tell him the problems. I thought Dr. Lohmann needed to know so he could be my advocate. It had seemed to me that every doctor Mother ever went to told the nurses how things *had to be*. I just assumed that was part of the role of a doctor. I was confounded when Bill would come back and say, "Well, Dr. Lohmann said they're doing just fine, Sue."

Who was Bill to believe? I never doubted that he loved me and was very concerned, but I also knew he would want to be very businesslike and not make ripples, because Bill Baier does not do that. Things go according to plan, and you don't upset people. You don't go against the rules.

"December 17: I should take her out of ICU."
—*from Bill's diary*

My own isolated world of fear was extended when Bill brought distressing news from Mary Helen and Max, our good friends from the Rio Grande Valley. Their daughter Cathy was hospitalized with serious injuries from an automobile accident. That was horrible.

Mary Helen and I went to SMU together, got married at the same time, and had our children together. Cathy was born just six months before Katherine, and she was like my own child. Our families grew up together. Now Cathy was also in her first year of college, at the University of Texas in Austin. It was break time for U.T., as it was for Vanderbilt, and Cathy was riding home from school with a friend when an oncoming truck pulled into the wrong lane. The young man she was riding with was killed.

I was stunned. Here was this child, like my own. . . . Such a routine trip, and now. . . . I felt the fear Mary Helen and Max must be experiencing. And I could do nothing to help—nothing but pray for Cathy and for the family of the boy who died. What a terrible Christmas theirs would be.

Hours and days plodded on, lonely and frustrating. Bill never failed—he came three times a day. The girls came when they could, but they were busy with party preparations. I was determined that their lives be normal, not locked into this ICU world. While the days were interminable, I dreaded most the evenings after Bill left, especially if there were no other visitors.

More people were coming now, and their visits meant more than they could imagine. Just a little time not to be alone. Each visitor made the time special—sometimes sad, other times happy—but always the memories that lingered helped relieve my desperation.

As Chickie and Hans walked up to my bed, thankful tears came. The sight of them flooded my mind with happy memories. Chickie and I were such close friends for so long. We graduated from SMU at the same time and shared an apartment until we both decided to move back home with our families. Chickie was the youngest of six children—much younger than her brothers and sisters. Her parents missed the bustling house, so they often asked me to come to Houston and spend weekends with Chickie and them.

In fact, the first time I went out with Bill, I was staying at her home. Chickie's father now assumed the role with me, standing there in his marvelous, old-fashioned way, checking out this Bill Baier. Thank goodness, Bill passed inspection. Chickie was my maid of honor when Bill and I were married.

Over the years, the four of us became very close friends. I was even comfortable tonight about Hans seeing me. Most men didn't seem able to handle looking at me in this condition, but I could relax with Hans. He was a friend, and we'd been through a great deal together.

Chickie was busy moistening a washcloth to wipe my face. "We had a letter from Oma, today," Hans said. "She wanted us to be sure to greet you."

Oma was Mrs. Flick, Hans's mother, who lived in Holland. We met her at Hans and Chickie's wedding, but I got to know her well on our first trip to The Hague. Although she spoke very little English, that didn't matter. She was one of those marvelous people you can understand and relate to without language.

She told Bill not to worry about me while he was at his conference; she was going to take care of me. The first day I was there, Mrs. Flick took me into a little Dutch bookstore and asked the owner for two small dictionaries. They were red, about one-and-a-half by two inches. And she wanted both English-Dutch and Dutch-English, in case she and I got into trouble. At the time, America's space program was getting a good deal of publicity, and she told the shopkeeper that I was from Houston, Texas. He was a delightful little bald man who spoke no English, and he became very excited and exclaimed, "Aha! Space City, USA." Each day after that, she showed up at the hotel, put her arm through mine, and off we went.

Two years later, when we moved to Holland, Mrs. Flick became our grandmother, our Oma, for the year. She said her family and ours were in America, so she would be our Oma.

"She's very excited and determined about coming for the holidays," Chickie said. "She'll be here in about two weeks."

"Of course, we'll bring her to see you," Hans added.

Both Hans and Chickie tried to mask the sadness in their eyes.

Before I got sick, we learned that Oma had cancer. She was coming to America for Christmas, one last trip. And our families were to be together again for a big, wonderful visit. We were all concerned about her malignancy and how we were going to handle getting through the holidays, knowing that we might never see her again.

Hand squeezes replaced talk as they stood on each side of my bed, searching for words. There were none. Surely they were wondering—as I was—how my illness would affect Oma. I hoped they did not see the tears in my eyes. Such hopes for happy times now filled with so much sadness. It didn't seem right. I didn't want to be an extra burden on Oma.

I felt it! A muscle above the front of my knee twitched, and I had made it happen! I was so excited. Every day I'd been taking inventory of my body. I was convinced that if I thought long enough and hard enough about moving, some day I would be able to do it. While I lay by myself, bored and desperate, tired of counting the tiny holes in the acoustical ceiling tile, I worked again and again to flex my muscles. Throughout the day, every day, I tested myself. Surely something had to start moving. Finally, it happened, and what a relief! Even though Bill had repeatedly reassured me, and I believed him, this was the real affirmation I needed. Here we go! Recovery is coming. I could hardly wait to show Bill.

Leg. Watch, Bill. See it move.

He studied the leg without knowing what to look for.

Moves. Over and over I made the muscle twitch until he saw it.

"Hey, it does move! Do it again." Gladly. Another demonstration for my beaming husband.

"Anything else moving?"

No. His smile dimmed ever so slightly. So did my enthusiasm. But this was a beginning, I told myself. That's what we needed— a start.

But I found it hard to cope with my disappointment and frustration when days passed and nothing else moved. I was so sure that things would go quickly once they started. Yet days went by, and, try as I might, there was no movement but that one twitching leg muscle.

One morning Bill stood quietly at the foot of the bed. There was the smile I fell in love with, the sparkle in his eyes. Slowly he raised his hand, and in it was a single Tiffany rose in a bud vase. Tears filled my eyes, but inside I was a huge, beaming smile. He set the vase where I could see it on the nightstand. I wished I could tell him how much I loved him for bringing this particular rose for me today.

After Bill and I were married, I began hinting that no one had ever given me roses, particularly long-stemmed roses—a dozen red ones. For years I kept after him, until I finally caught on that hinting to Bill Baier about something you want is the best way *not* to get it. He likes to surprise me, not to be told what I want. Finally, one Valentine's Day, Bill gave me six rose bushes. He was still not buying me the ones with long stems, but I was to have roses. One plant actually was a tree—it was a Tiffany rose. The blossoms are pale pink with a yellow center, and the fragrance is magnificent. This one flower had more meaning than anything from a florist shop. Each time I looked at it, I saw Bill's smile again.

I hoped the staff wouldn't notice the rose. I was so afraid it would be taken away, like the poinsettia Sally had sent last week. That nearly broke my heart. Bill had brought in a beautiful poinsettia from my high school friend. How were we to know live plants weren't allowed in ICU? The plant was there two days before anyone noticed—or acknowledged that they noticed. All of a sudden, a nurse stormed indignantly into my cubicle and snatched up my poinsettia. "What's this doing in here? You know you can't have this in ICU." I was startled and upset. If it had been there for two days and not done any harm, why was it wrong now?

Everyone apparently decided to overlook the one rose next to my bed, and Bill continued to bring me a fresh one every few days until the frost ended the season.

Before the regular staff left for the holidays, there was much talk about the hospital party. The day of the party, I watched Vickie happily move from bed to bed, caring for her patients. Though she wasn't my nurse, Vickie waved to me and spoke each time she passed. After work, she changed clothes at the hospital and was ready to go to the party. I watched her putting on her jewelry and modeling her dress for the evening-shift nurses. She said she was going alone, and I wondered why her husband wasn't going with her—they were newly married. The staff was all talk about who was going to the party—husbands, wives, and dates. It made me sad that Vickie was going alone. You just didn't go to a couples Christmas party without your husband.

It's none of your business, Sue, I told myself. But still it troubled me. I wouldn't go to such a party without Bill. It wouldn't be any fun. Oh, how I'd love to go to a party with Bill tonight.

Instead, all I could do was lie here in this miserable heat and perspire. My nameless day nurse had bundled me up with covers before going off duty. I felt worse than on any August day I could remember, and I remembered a lot of them.

Even as a young girl, I always dreaded the summer heat. I stayed wet all summer. We got our first air-conditioning when I was in ninth grade. We had moved to the country, into a new home that had two window units. That was magnificent! Daddy also had the house built with an attic fan. Even on the hottest summer nights, we could turn off the air-conditioning, open the windows, and let the attic fan create a cooling breeze in every room. That's what I needed now, a fan—and to get rid of these covers.

Since Daddy owned an automobile dealership, we also had one of the first air-conditioned cars. I was fifteen, and that was sheer luxury! Plastic pipes ran from the rear window and fit the curvature of the back of the car. It was quite a contraption. As soon as we got the car, we left on a family trip to California. Daddy was excited because we could cross the desert in an air-conditioned car. Of course it rained all the way across the desert, and the air-conditioning froze up. We pulled into a service station, and nobody in that part of the country had ever seen such a thing. It was a small town, and people came running from all over to look at the amazing car. But no one knew what was wrong with it—or how to make it work again.

In spite of having an air-conditioned house and car, school was another matter. I perspired most of May through September. My hair was always wet, and I could do nothing about it. I just dripped. None of the other girls seemed to be as soaked as I was. People used to say it was healthy to perspire in the heat, but it embarrassed me miserably. It still does. Even in my cubicle, I hated looking wet and sweaty all the time. Would I *ever* get these nurses to leave the covers off?

Bill had developed an organized plan of attack to get the house cleaned for the girls' party. As the invitation replies came in, so did the offers of help from mothers of the invited guests. I was very grateful, although I'm sure Bill wondered what he would do with these volunteers during the party.

Gerda and Wim also offered to help. They were a Dutch couple in Houston on the same exchange program that had taken us to Holland. They came to the hospital every week to see me. The first time, I was amazed at how they took this whole ICU experience in stride. Then Gerda told of being very ill in Holland, so she was quite familiar with intensive care. They both inspected all my equipment and pronounced it to be excellent. When they heard from Bill about the party, they were anxious to be involved. Gerda wanted to bring food, and they both volunteered to help in the kitchen. They weren't quite sure just what kind of party this was, but they were determined to be a part of it—and to help Bill.

Everyone was pitching in. Some girls from one of Elizabeth's school clubs came to the house, wished her a Merry Christmas, and gave her poinsettias for party decorations. The next day, other friends of hers brought a Christmas tree and asked if they could come back later and decorate it. Bill was overwhelmed. So were Elizabeth and I. The girls returned on several nights and made cookies and decorated the tree and the house.

I was sure Bill still would have liked to cancel the party and all the bother it was causing him, but he seemed to understand what a lift it was giving me. I was so pleased that things were falling into place. Even what little involvement I had with the party helped me face the empty feeling of Christmas in a hospital.

The night was bleak. I watched the window across the room, and I saw flashes of lightning. It was disconcerting. What if the power went out? Was there definitely a backup system to keep my respirator going? It's not that I mind rain. I enjoy a rainy day, being home alone, feeling snug and secure. That's the perfect time to tackle a closet or a chest of drawers—to restore order where it has been overlooked. Rainy evenings with everyone home are mellow times. The patter of rain is soothing, a sound of cleansing, of tranquility. I wanted to be home now. I wanted to sit with Bill and smile over each flash of light, each clap of thunder. I wanted to smell the fresh pine of the Christmas tree and the garlands by the hearth—and watch burning logs crackle in the fireplace. I wanted Bill.

But there was nothing to smell, even if I were able now. There were no logs, no fire—just the citrus-yellow ICU wall crowned with sagging garlands. Then suddenly the garish world was softened and freshened by the warm smile of Mary, a neighbor and friend. Mary and her family, which most notably included a daughter, Jane, moved into our subdivision the same week we did, and their daughter and Elizabeth started off to first grade together.

Elizabeth came home her first day very excited. "I have a new friend. Her name is Jane, but her middle name is Elizabeth, and her daddy works at the same place my daddy does. And they live here, too." Some time later, I met Mary in the builder's office, and we became friends almost immediately. Our daughters are still best friends, and Bill had told me that Jane was at the house almost every night lately, helping Elizabeth and Katherine.

"Jane says your girls are doing a wonderful job with organizing," Mary reported. "Of course, Jane is right in the thick of it."

Yes. Mary smiled recognition of my response. Jane or Elizabeth must have explained spelling to Mary.

Helping.

"I'm not sure how much she's helping, but she's certainly cheering them on."

Tonight Mary could fill me in on school and neighborhood news. Bill always felt we had more important things to deal with during his limited time, so I missed hearing the local happenings. Mary had been so busy since taking a full-time job that her gift of this visit was all the more generous. I hoped she would find time to come again—and she did. Very quietly, she would just show up at the nicest times. Actually, it was she who made the times nice.

The weekend of the party arrived. I concentrated on last-minute details, spelling and checking them with Bill. He took my questions and unfailingly reported back that yes, the girls had done this or that. Meanwhile, he was also checking his own lists with me, such items as vacuuming and cleaning the bathrooms. When the girls came, we talked about last-minute food preparation and about what they should wear.

What would I wear if I were going to be home? What did it matter? I couldn't be there.

"December 20: Wreaths on doors. Party guest book. Load camera."

—from Bill's diary

Saturday, December 20. The big day. Mother came to the hospital early in the morning. She and Bill had decided previously that if she visited me on Saturday mornings, he could sleep in and not have to rush to the hospital. I liked the idea, because on weekdays she always came at the same time as Bill.

On Saturday Mother could be alone with me and have time to share all the girl-talk news I missed.

This morning, though, was a little awkward. We both were thinking about the girls' party, and Mother had not changed her mind about being involved. I wished I could talk to her, to make her understand. There was still time. She could still go to the house today and be part of the fun. She would love it. They would all be so glad to see her. But that wasn't going to happen. There was no point in spoiling this time with her by thinking such thoughts.

Mother, however, came prepared with a distraction. She pulled a cluster of pedicure equipment from her purse. "Your toenails need clipping. I thought this would be a good time to do that." She started working on them. "Do you know you have calluses on the bottom of your feet?" I knew, but I certainly hadn't had the opportunity to notice them for several weeks. "I brought a pumice stone today. I can just take off a little each week, and by the time you're up again, they'll all be gone."

It felt wonderful to have Mother's caressing hands working on my feet, and it was good to hear her news of the Bridge Club and family friends.

Whenever Mother and I were together, we always shared memories of our beautiful tour of Scandinavia the previous fall. Today was no exception.

After Daddy died, Mother asked me to take a trip with her. She had been tied down for so long. She hadn't even taken a weekend off to go see my brother in Dallas because she wouldn't leave Houston and Daddy. Earlier in her life, opportunities for travel were limited by her work in the family business. Beyond a few family vacations, Mother's only real adventure had been coming to Holland to visit us. And that had given her a taste for travel.

I had never traveled without Bill, but he felt I should go with her. Mother needed a trip and she needed me with her. I thought perhaps she was considering Colorado, or some other interesting place in the United States. She always said there was so much to see in America without traveling to other countries.

Then one day she phoned, very excited. "I have always dreamed of going to Scandinavia, and I've found a nice tour. Could we do that?" My heavens, I hadn't expected Europe!

Bill thought it was wonderful. He'd been to Norway on business and loved the country. "Because of the circumstances, and since I've been there, I think just this once it would be a very special thing for you and your mother to do."

We went in October and had a glorious two weeks.

Now Mother's eyes welled with tears as she said, "Oh, Sue, I'm so happy we had that trip together before. . . ." Her voice trailed off and she concentrated on the pumice stone.

There was no mention of the girls' party, but I understood. Instead, she talked of cherries and olives. This was a little tradition she shared with the girls. When they were small, Mother always put green cherries in the bottoms of their glasses to encourage them to drink their milk. Anyone else would have used red cherries, but not Mother. She used green. Somewhere along the way, she also discovered that they loved black olives. And those, too, became special. So, at Christmas, ever since they were toddlers, Nana has placed under the tree a little jar of green cherries and a little can of black olives for each of them.

"Should I do it this year, Sue?"

Yes.

"It seems rather silly now. Maybe they're getting too old. Do you think they would miss them if I just skipped that this year?"

Yes. The girls cherish all our traditions and would be brokenhearted if she dropped the custom. This year, more than any other, they needed to continue the traditions.

I checked the patch of window across the room. Twilight came early at this time of year. In spirit I was home with everyone getting ready for the guests. Last year, we'd had a brunch, but this year we chose early evening, six-to-eight, for a buffet. That way, the sixty-some guests would be free to go on to other parties.

I watched the time and imagined the flurry of last-minute

activity at home. I could even feel the countdown. I hoped Bill would remember to have all the girls sign the guest book at the front door. And photographs . . . would he remember to put film in the camera?

The party time arrived and so did Margie, without explanation. She and Bill must have decided that she would keep me company this evening. I don't think that she even mentioned the party, but we both knew that she was there to be with me, and I was grateful. She stayed a long time. Perhaps the staff also realized how badly I needed company tonight. Or they were relieved to have someone as capable as Margie staying with me for a while. When she came for her regular Wednesday noon visits, Bill was always there and time was limited. This was the first time she and I had been alone in ages. She talked about Archie and the children and friends here and in The Hague. And about the good times in Holland.

"Remember Gerry?"

Could not forget.

"I had a letter from her this week. She asked about you— wanted to know whether you still have your same white car." Margie was grinning broadly. She must have been able to see me smiling inside at the mention of Gerry. This marvelous Dutch woman made an art of international hospitality and was determined to take care of all of us foreign guests in Holland.

Bill and I had bought a white station wagon to drive while we were in Europe. Driving in The Hague is something of a challenge. Many of the American women wouldn't try, and even some of the Dutch women exclaimed, "Sue! You're driving in town!" But there were school activities I just wouldn't miss. Once I learned to handle the traffic, I had few problems. I just began driving like one of the locals. At all but the main intersections, traffic coming from the right has the right of way. All of the streets are full of bicycles and motorcycles. Government taxes make cars very expensive for the Dutch to buy, so they use two-wheeled transportation and zip up and down the street in front of you and at both sides. Driving in the middle, with all the bicycles, is quite an experience. But I was determined. Keeping moving is the challenge. A milk cart will stop in the middle of a tiny, narrow street, and it might sit there for a half hour before the milkman returns, so you just drive up over the curb and keep on going. I did my share of those maneuvers during the year.

But traffic was not the problem the day Gerry and I went to a flower show in a little village out in the countryside. I picked her up and we headed out of the city. She is a funny, jovial, very happy person—even when issuing driving instructions. We had a wonderful time at the flower show and then returned to my car, which would not start. We were out in the middle of nowhere. But Gerry said, "Not to worry." Without a pause, she was out of the car and hiking down the road. I felt terrible, because it was a warm day and she was a large woman—and probably a good ten years older than I. As she marched off, she told me to sit there and wait. Eventually she reappeared with a man in a service-station truck. I learned later that when she got to the station, which was a fair distance down the road, the attendant told her he couldn't go with her. He was the only one at the station and he insisted, "I can't close the station." But Gerry would not be put off. She eyed him squarely and said, "She's a *visitor* to Holland. Think of the image we're sending." So he came.

He started the car with no difficulty, and soon we were on our way home again, with Gerry assuring me, "He did it because you're a guest in our country."

Toward the end of our stay in Holland, I walked out of a shop near Gerry's home and found a paper stuck in my windshield wiper. It looked official, but I had no idea what it said. I didn't know enough Dutch to read all the traffic signs, but I recognized most of the negative ones. I'd parked in this lot before, but I looked around for something that indicated that I'd violated a law. I could see nothing different.

So I showed the paper to Gerry. "What do I have?" She shot through the ceiling. "They have changed that to a pay parking lot just this week, but the sign is hidden," she said. "You drive me over there."

I must admit I was concerned about the ticket. We were just

getting ready to leave the country, and we didn't need a parking violation, especially after going all year without any problems.

Gerry marched up to the parking lot attendant and gave him a lecture. "You knew by looking at her license plate that she was a visitor here," she accused. She was right. There were special plates to identify cars of foreigners. "You *knew* that, and you *knew* you'd just changed this to a pay lot this week and that she probably couldn't read the sign that's hidden partially behind a tree where nobody can see it." His face showed embarrassment. "So, you just tear up this ticket right now." And she was so intimidating that, without a word, he *did*!

Margie knew we no longer had that station wagon, but thinking about those days was the best distraction I could have this evening. I was so grateful she had been here to help me through this lonely time.

After the party, Bill came immediately to the hospital to show me the Polaroid pictures he'd taken throughout the evening. I cherished each image, wanting to hear everything. Bill tried to remember the names of all the girls who were there. He told about Bess, about Gerda and Wim, and Carolyn, one of the mothers—all working in the kitchen.

"Gerda brought a fish-shaped mousse and a dessert," he said. "The mousse was so pretty the girls didn't want to cut into it and destroy it."

Our girls?

"No, the guests," he said. He was smiling contentedly. "Elizabeth finally cut a piece, and everyone said it and the dessert were delicious. Gerda and Wim seemed to enjoy watching all the excitement."

Bill assured me that everything had gone very well, and that when Katherine and Elizabeth came tomorrow, they would fill me in on details he'd forgotten. I could tell he was tired—and very, very glad it was over. But I was so happy it had happened. I *had* been right in insisting that the party go on. Life, indeed, must continue for the girls. I was so proud of them both for being able to do it—and happy for them that this was a night they would never forget.

I thought about Bess, Carolyn, Wim, and Gerda—in the kitchen all evening. How was I ever going to thank them for helping to make it work? And Bill, dear Bill. He had done all this for me. What did I ever do to deserve you, Bill Baier? My heart was bursting with love.

9

"December 21: Hospital called 3 P.M. Overdose. Coma!"
—*from Bill's diary*

Bill arrived after church. How was I to explain to him what was happening to me?

When I woke in the morning, my tongue was curled over and back, caught rigidly between my upper and lower teeth on the left side of my mouth. I couldn't control the muscles of my jaw or tongue, so I was biting my tongue, and it hurt terribly. Even when I was turned, it couldn't slide free; it was locked in by my teeth.

Carol was on duty that morning, and I tried to spell the problem to her, but she misunderstood. "Don't worry, Sue, you won't swallow your tongue." I couldn't get through to her that I was biting myself. So many words to spell when I was in such pain. And today she had too many patients to wait for further spelling. The more frantically I tried to communicate, the more she assured me that everything was all right.

Dr. Lohmann came in. I was sure he'd do something for me if I could just explain it to him. But, as always, when I tried to signal him with my eyes, he turned away. "Oh, nurse," he said to the closest one, "see what she wants." And he left. The nurse was new in the unit. She looked at me, shrugged, and walked off.

Immediately after the doctor left, Bill came from church. What a blessing. I signaled urgently.

Find Lohmann. We must catch him before he leaves the hospital. Bill turned to Carol as she passed the cubicle and asked, "Has Dr. Lohmann been in?"

"It's his day off," she answered and hurried away. I couldn't believe she had not seen him.

Lohmann here. Find.

"Sue, I've told you that it's his day off. There's no way we can reach him. You just don't do that to a doctor." There was irritation in Bill's voice.

Tongue.

"I know, Sue. On my way in, Carol told me you were concerned. But she said you can't swallow it."

Hurts.

Bill could see I was upset, but still he didn't understand. I couldn't get through to him. Finally, he refused to continue.

"Sue, let's just drop the subject. This is going to upset you; it's going to upset me. Let's just forget about Dr. Lohmann."

The frustration was devastating. I had just seen the man! Bill asked Carol if there was anything she could do. She said she would try to reach whoever was covering for Dr. Lohmann.

By now I was terribly agitated from the pain and exasperation. Bill could see it in my eyes, but he felt helpless, so he decided it was best for him to leave. And he did.

His departure was devastating. Tears gushed. I felt abandoned. What can I do now? Bill's gone, and I'm all alone with no one to speak for me. Why couldn't he understand?

But Carol was still there. Please, Carol, understand me. She came in as soon as Bill left. Again I spelled.

Tongue . . . teeth . . . hurts.

For a moment, she silently mouthed the words, still not comprehending. She looked in my mouth, her expression remaining puzzled. But she did sense something serious was wrong.

"All right, Sue. I'll try to get something to help you."

The doctor on call diagnosed the problem: a swollen tongue from a reaction to the antibiotics. If they cut down the antibiotics, the swelling eventually would subside and the problem would be corrected. But since I was so upset now, he ordered an injection of Benadryl to reduce the swelling faster.

Carol handled the injection carefully. She gave such easy shots. I relaxed, knowing I would feel better soon. But suddenly I felt very strange. I could not see anything!

I heard people's voices—in fact, I could hear *everything* that was being said. I heard nurses rushing breathlessly, and asking, "Oh, my goodness, what's happened?" I felt them taking my pulse and blood pressure. More voices. "What's happened to her? What's wrong?"

"Benadryl. She's reacting." That was Carol. I knew her voice. It was firm and steady. "Keep watching her blood pressure." The blood-pressure cuff was pumped up again. More voices. The routine sounds of ICU seemed louder, distorted. So much commotion around me.

I was in a tunnel. I could vaguely see something round and I had the sensation of falling. I was slipping away. But then I heard Carol's voice close to me, steady and clear. . . .

"Sue, that shot I gave you apparently was too strong. You're overreacting to it. Your vital signs are good." She spoke slowly, intently, directly to me. "You stick with us, and we're going to take care of you. You will be all right, I promise you. You're going to make it."

I believed her. Her voice was so convincing. But I also knew I must fight to stay alert. And fight I did.

The radio was on. The Houston Oilers were playing Pittsburgh, a play-off game. Bill and I always followed the games and all the players—especially Earl Campbell, who was doing so well this season. I made myself listen to that ball game and keep up with every play. Come on, Earl!

"Come on, Sue, wake up. Open your eyes." It was Bill's voice over the sound of the radio. "Katherine and Elizabeth are here. You've got to open your eyes."

He had both girls with him and he was calling me, repeatedly begging me to open my eyes. My mind fought to react. I was frightened. If Bill is back already—and has both girls with him—this must be serious. But I'm all right, Bill.

"Sue, Sue, open your eyes." His voice was close and intense. "Wake up, Sue, wake up." I just couldn't make my eyes open. But I did fight to keep my mind on that football game. I couldn't let go of that game. The Oilers and I were fighting together to win.

I don't know what time I pulled back out again. When I finally opened my eyes ever so slightly, the girls were gone but Bill was still there, talking to me, trying to make me wake up. I felt myself slipping away again. He shook me, gently but very earnestly. "Sue, you've got to stay awake." I forced my eyes open again and again.

Just briefly I caught a glimpse of Phil's white uniform at the foot of my bed. Carol must have gone off duty; Phil's on the second shift. Thinking was laborious. Then I felt excruciating pain. Phil was jamming the head of an IV tube into the top of my foot, the bony part of the foot. I will never forget the stab of that needle. I thought I was going to leave the bed. I tried to open my eyes, but they were flooded with tears. Don't you know I can feel? How could you do that to me? Dear God, help me!

Bill kept talking to me, forcing my attention onto the football game, trying to keep me alert. Finally, the game was over. The Oilers and I had won! I saw in Bill's eyes the mixture of relief and sadness. I understand why you left, Bill. It was just a misunderstanding and it's all right. You're here now and that is all that matters. I wanted to spell all that to him, but my eyes were too full—and I couldn't find the energy. Some other time, Bill, I can tell you. Now all I can do is love you. Obviously the staff was allowing Bill to stay longer, probably until I was fully awake. I basked in these wonderful minutes with Bill beside me, tenderly holding my hands.

Only when Aurilla appeared to take my vital signs and turn me did the mood evaporate. This was the nurse I felt the least empathy from. And now, after the traumatic day I'd had, she was to be my night nurse. Who assigns these people? I cringed inside when she touched me. How could I explain this woman to Bill? I had wanted him to see her in action, to see how roughly she treated me. I wanted him to see why I felt I was just an object to be tended.

Very abruptly, Aurilla turned me, right in front of Bill, shoving the pillows harshly into my back. Did he see that? Did he realize how miserable it was to be lumped like a sack of potatoes? And what could he do about her, even if he did understand?

Bill stayed well beyond the evening visiting hours. It was the longest time I'd been with him in nearly three weeks. I wished I could tell him that in spite of Aurilla, it was a very special time for me. But finally he had to go.

Again loneliness—until Ginnie came for my range-of-motion therapy. Charles had trained her to work with me as he did, and she was a delight. I especially enjoyed her regular Sunday night visits.

"Hi. Sorry I'm so late," she said. "Time got away from me." As she talked, she was already working my fingers and right arm, and her voice rang with laughter. I was glad she was late. If she'd come much earlier, before I was fully awake, they'd have sent her away.

Rob? I spelled her husband's name. It troubled me that Ginnie had to work Sunday nights. She should be able to stay home with her new husband on Sundays. It wasn't fair that she should have to work all week and then weekends, too.

"I've parked Rob and our bags of dirty clothes over at the laundromat again." Ginnie always understood my spelling perfectly, and she always talked to me, including me in her life away from the hospital. She saw a question in my eyes before I could spell it—even while she was moving to my legs and feet. "Don't worry. Rob doesn't mind. He's good at laundry." I loved her laughter. I was so glad to have her here.

When she finished, she leaned over and said, "See you tomorrow," in a cute little whisper, as if this were a secret. In fact, none of the staff seemed to notice she'd been here.

Bill's chores never ran out these last few days before Christmas. The car Elizabeth drove needed new tires, he reported, and I reminded him that Katherine had an appointment with the orthodontist. Funny how I remembered that. And Christmas cards still flooded in, with Bill hurriedly addressing the responses every day. Plus there were Christmas presents.

At the top of the gift list were the girls. In October, I had bought Katherine and Elizabeth Scandinavian charms, which I had tucked away for Christmas. Now I was glad I had them. And there were some other gifts already purchased. For graduation last spring we gave Katherine luggage. At the time, we bought the complete set, reserving some of the pieces for Christmas. Elizabeth was to go on her first ski trip December 28 with her Young Life group. She'd counted on this for months, and Bill and I agreed that, of course, she should go. In November, she and I had shopped for her ski clothes. We bought everything except the *après-ski* boots and a few small things. So Bill and I reviewed what she had and what she still needed.

Bill looked up from his notes. "Who's going to pay for all these ski clothes?" He was just beginning to see how much daughters cost!

She half. We half for Christmas. He made a note of the split arrangement. I could see this was not going over too well, but he said nothing. He would send her out to buy what she needed.

For years our girls had exchanged Christmas ornaments with their cousins, Mary and Ann, in Maine. The four of them were acquiring nice collections. This fall, at a church bazaar, I bought some little wooden sleigh ornaments and had the cousins' names printed on them. I spelled to Bill what they were and where they were stored, so he could wrap them and mail them off to Maine. He was becoming practiced at being patient with my requests. He just nodded when I told him about buying a wedding gift for our next-door neighbor, Julie, who was getting married two days after Christmas. A bridal registry simplified that.

Mother once mentioned needing a new watch that she could read more easily since her eye surgery. I knew Bill would not want to shop for that, so I spelled to him to give her a check toward the watch and promise her I would shop for it with her when I was better. This was going to be a terrible Christmas for Mother, her first since Daddy died. Having all the family together would have been especially important this year. I wished I could do more than a promissory gift.

Fortunately, I'd been to several Christmas bazaars, so I had purchased more gifts than usual ahead of time. They were hidden in different places—squirreled away in a box under another box in a closet, or in some other obscure location—in hopes that the girls wouldn't find them. It was terribly involved spelling out all these gifts and their hiding places, but at least I remembered where everything was.

I had to rely on the girls to buy my gift for Bill. I sent them shopping for an electric shaver.

There was one little gift for Bill that I could not forget. At the November meeting of my Zeta sorority chapter, the owner of a good men's store had displayed gift ideas for husbands. Several items became door prizes. He gave away a tie and a shoeshine kit, two or three little things. Naturally, I didn't win anything; I never do. Finally he announced two gift certificates. I sat there thinking, wouldn't it be funny if I won one of these? And lo and behold, for the second certificate he called out, "Sue Baier!"

The certificate was tucked away for Bill, all ready to be slipped into his stocking on Christmas Eve. But now I had to spell out its hiding place so he could dig it out. Even Santa couldn't plan any surprises for Bill.

The girls would get their father his usual jar of peanuts—and he must have his Aramis Duck, a special shower soap they loved giving him.

The countdown for Christmas was moving in earnest. I am sure I was more intent on it than Bill. It was obvious he—and Mother—would prefer to skip the holidays this year. But I was determined: there would be Christmas.

On December 22, per my instructions, Bill moved the turkey from the freezer into the refrigerator. Thank goodness I'd bought one right after Thanksgiving. One less thing for Bill to shop for now.

Much as I tried to make Christmas my total preoccupation, I was haunted by fear after the overdose of Benadryl. Two days later, Bill finally talked to Dr. Lohmann about the Benadryl— which had relaxed my tongue by the time I awoke completely. When the hospital called Bill on Sunday, they'd said I was in a coma. But now Dr. Lohmann said I had been in no danger. Everything was fine. He'd talked to the nurses. I wondered whether he had talked with Carol.

"Don't worry, she's being well taken care of," Bill quoted. The Benadryl dosage I was given, Dr. Lohmann assured him, was comparable to taking two aspirin instead of one.

I wanted to ask Bill if he remembered warning the staff when I was admitted that I had a low tolerance for such medications. I'd watched the nurse write the notation. Specifically, I was not to be given more than one aspirin. But it was just too many words to spell.

I was no longer afraid of the disease, but of the system.

I could see Bill's frustration. His face showed his doubt. Who was he to believe? Was he beginning to sense that something was inconsistent? Yet Lohmann was a doctor, a person in authority. If he stopped trusting my doctor, what else did he have to go on? And always, Bill believed, one had to get along. Making trouble was counterproductive. Besides, he could see I was still very ill. He must have wondered if it was getting to me, just lying there day after day with nothing to do. How could he know what was real and what was imagined? Oh, Bill, I am not imagining these problems.

Frantically, I spelled to him. *No sleep . . . . Tests . . . . Pain . . . . Lights . . . . Need signal for attention.* He wrote every word, with patience. He would see what he could do.

With Katherine back in town and Elizabeth on vacation, I finally had some time with my daughters. They came separately to tell me all about the party, their friends, their plans. Katherine had a date this week with a young man from Vanderbilt. I always knew everyone the girls went out with, but not this young man. Though she was eighteen and away from home, I was still concerned about whom she would be with, and I longed to meet him. The following day I listened to her description of the evening. They'd had a good time, and he asked her to go out to dinner with him and his parents on New Year's Eve. New Year's Eve—and to an elegant hotel dining room. Normally, I didn't like the girls being out on New Year's Eve, but this would be just five minutes from our home. Besides, they would be with his parents. Even though I did not know them, it should certainly be all right.

It was good that this reasoning rambled in my thoughts. Of course Katherine did not need to ask permission; she was a college student. But mothers never stop being concerned about their daughters.

My girls' frequent visits reminded me of Cathy, still hospitalized from that dreadful accident. I could imagine what she and her parents had been going through. Bill had talked with Max and was assured that Cathy was doing well—under the circumstances. How difficult this must be for Max, a doctor, to wait out the recovery of his own daughter. Since I'd gotten sick, Max had given Bill so much support. Bill often called him for reassurances and explanations of my condition, and he always seemed to feel better after their conversations.

I worried about Cathy and I especially wished I could be with Mary Helen, to share her burden. But I could be of no help now to my friends—or to anyone.

Christmas Eve came too quickly. I wasn't ready. I still couldn't accept the idea that I would not be home with my family.

In the morning, Bill stopped at the office to water his plant before coming to the hospital. I was waiting impatiently for him. More lists. I had to stay mentally busy. I ran through the menu. They were to have turkey and dressing—everything. There was a packaged cornbread stuffing mix that we all liked, and it was very easy to prepare if they followed the directions. They must have sweet potatoes, though they'd probably use the canned ones, topped with marshmallows. I always made a gelatin salad.

"No," Bill said. "I'm not going to fool with all that." They would just have spiced peaches.

Appetizers and desserts were no problem. They had received so many Christmas goodies.

We finished with the menu and moved on to last-minute gifts. Suddenly that morning I'd remembered our niece Mary's birthday. Bill's sister, Barbara, and I decided years ago that we lived too far apart to know what the girls liked or wanted. We just send checks for all birthdays.

That reminded Bill he hadn't mailed our usual Christmas checks to his parents. With them, too, it was hard knowing what they could use, so our custom was to send money for something special. I was sorry these remembrances would be late, but I knew they would understand how busy Bill was now. He wasn't too busy, however, for one more special thoughtfulness this morning. Elizabeth had noticed that my legs needed shaving, so Bill had brought my shaver. Before going off with his list of last-minute errands, he shaved my legs and underarms.

As he left, my mind was still racing. Had we covered everything? What else should I be remembering? When he blew a kiss and waved good-bye, I suddenly knew it just didn't matter. There was nothing I could do now to help make Christmas happen—or to stop it from coming. Now my world felt very, very empty.

Early on Christmas Eve night, the three of them came—Bill, Katherine, and Elizabeth—wearing their bravest smiles and carrying a tiny plastic Christmas tree, about eight inches tall, bedecked with little bows. After the poinsettia experience, Bill knew they couldn't bring in anything live, except the roses he continued to smuggle in.

It was so thoughtful of them to bring this little tree, but so sad. I've always disliked artificial trees because they don't smell like pine, so we always put up real trees, with all the mess that accompanied them. This little plastic tree was almost too much for me to bear. I fought back the tears and tried to show a smile in my eyes.

Thank you. Spelling was easier tonight than spoken words would have been. The lump in my throat didn't show.

Bill and the girls were due at Maurice and Nancy's for dinner at seven o'clock. That would be nice for them, a good break from the somberness of home and the hospital. Maurice, an old friend of Bill's from Rice, was from Houston. His parents had always been good to Bill, treating him like a son, since his own parents lived so far away. They'd also invited Mother, but she didn't know them well. Tonight she preferred being with a close friend of hers. It was going to be a rough Christmas Eve for her—for all of my family.

Bill was looking at his watch. This visit had to be brief, but I wanted them never to leave. I tried not to let their dinner invitation bother me, but it did. I was being selfish, but tonight I couldn't control my feelings. I felt left out, cheated.

The night was bad. The third-shift respiratory therapist was from an agency and not good at all. He wanted to be helpful and he was friendly enough, but his suctioning never helped me. I still felt full every time he finished.

If he was a frustration, nursing care that night was worse. I was assigned to Louise, a nurse who didn't seem able to deal well with the English language, which created a problem when it came to spelling. She meant well, but she just kept saying, "What do you want? What do you want?" There was no way to communicate with her.

"Maybe you want to turn." When turning me, she repeatedly asked if it was all right, but she couldn't understand my response, and the harder she tried to position me comfortably, the worse it got. I have never been in such bizarre positions in my life. There was no way I would sleep this Christmas Eve with these two tending me. I just watched the clock and prayed for morning and the new shift.

At six-thirty, I felt we'd make it. But before the new crew made rounds, Louise returned, still determined to help me.

"Maybe your back hurts," she announced. "I'll give you a shot."

I reacted vehemently, but of course she didn't comprehend. Bill, Mother, and the girls would be here early this morning. I didn't want a shot that could knock me out. She paid no attention to my protestations and gave me the hypo. There was nothing I could do, nothing but fight sleep.

Minutes after the hypo, the respiratory therapist prepared to leave. On his way out, he walked past my bed, smiled, and said, "Merry Christmas!" This was the first time this season I'd heard the greeting, and I plummeted to the depths of dejection.

The morning staff made rounds and Louise announced that I was resting comfortably. At least the fury I felt helped me stay awake.

Soon, Bill, Mother, Elizabeth, and Katherine paraded in. On our fall trip, Mother and I had met a couple who carried automatic folding umbrellas that snapped open with the push of a button. Throughout the trip we fought with our pesky old umbrellas, repeatedly resolving to get one of those new models.

Now my beloved four walked up to my cubicle, all smiles, while Katherine extended a small umbrella. Suddenly she pushed the button, and up flew the open umbrella, as they all shouted, "Merry Christmas!"

Elizabeth was carrying a huge stuffed dog sent to me by a woman from the office at Lee High School. Bill held up a little shopping bag lined with pink tissue paper. In it were earrings that he and I had selected before I got sick. Mother, her eyes brimming with tears, stood patting my feet. Everyone was trying to be joyful, but this must have been the saddest sight in the world!

And what did I do? I immediately told Bill about Louise and the hypo. It was a downer for all of them. The brave, happy expressions drained from all four faces. I should have waited, but I thought maybe something could undo the shot if Bill knew. Of course, we both knew there was nothing to be done.

I hated what I'd done. Here they were, all wishing me Merry Christmas and trying so hard to be cheerful, and I ruined everything. I was the one who'd insisted this be a normal, happy Christmas for them. I'd put Bill through so much trying to make sure that everything could go on as always, and now what good cheer they'd managed to summon was trampled.

They stayed on, struggling to find things to say. Mother told me she was waiting until we could go shopping together to buy my Christmas present. She just couldn't do it now, she said. She bit her lip, obviously wishing to take back the words. Finally it was time for them to go home for breakfast and to put the turkey in the oven for dinner. Bill promised he'd be back after they got things started. They left, and my Christmas gifts went with them. They wanted to leave the stuffed dog, at least, but there was no room.

Tears gushed. I had won the battle against sleep, but I felt I'd lost everything else as I watched them leave. I'd wanted this to be a good Christmas for my family, but I killed it for them. Why was this happening to us? I prayed earnestly for this burden to be lifted from all of us. I didn't blame God for my illness, and I wasn't asking for a miracle. I just needed to know that this was going to end. Please, God, give us all the courage to make it through whatever lies ahead. *Our Father, who art in heaven.* . . .

The intensive care unit was nearly empty of patients. Everyone who could leave left before the holidays, and there were no new surgical patients. Surely no one who had a choice came in to the hospital for Christmas. Two smiling nurses walked into my cubicle and announced that I was their patient today. Like most of the others this week, they were strangers. I wondered what to expect.

"I'm Kathleen, and this is Judith." Kathleen had sparkling eyes and a great laugh.

"Hello, Sue. You look like you might like a bit of attention this morning. Would I be right?" Judith's smile was so warm and kind, and her voice was thick with a beautiful, rich Caribbean accent.

Yes. If only she could know how badly I needed attention. Or perhaps she did. As soon as they began talking, I knew these two were wonderful. Where did they come from?

"We are going to take care of you this morning," Kathleen announced, and I knew she meant it. They began my bath, talking to each other—and to me. They were friends, and both had volunteered to spend this day in ICU. Their friendship was evident from their easy banter. It was obvious they were caring women, as they tried to master my spelling. And they were very concerned about making me comfortable.

After a long and thorough bath, Kathleen asked, "Do they brush your teeth?" Aha! These are good nurses.

Yes.

Next they tried to figure out how to do it. It was fun listening to the two of them speculate on ways to accomplish the brushing. While they were trying to think of the alternatives and study the merits of each, they made it a little game. For most of the morning they created a distraction, doing what they could to get me through this difficult day.

A little later, after I'd rested a bit, Judith came back to the cubicle and stood looking down at me, smiling warmly. Gently she lifted my head and shoulders, cradling me in her full, brown arms with an easy rocking motion. Then, softly, she began to sing island lullabies to me. Her deep, resonant voice was so soothing and caressing. My tears ran freely, releasing much pain and sadness.

During the quiet times of that morning, I watched the clock and could envision the family at home. We had a special Christmas morning routine, established over the years—including the same breakfast menu I had as a child. With Mother there, I knew everything would go just right. She had welcomed the girls into the kitchen since they were little children, so they all worked together smoothly. How I would love to peek in on them, scurrying around the kitchen with breakfast and dinner all going at once.

When they returned in late morning and found me in better spirits, there was a look of relief on all their faces. Katherine and Elizabeth were wearing their charms as necklaces—how pretty they looked. They both were chattering away, telling me about all their gifts. Bill smiled at me—surely remembering, as I was doing, the early years when the girls rushed to tell us what Santa brought them.

Bill was also buoyed by Christmas phone calls. He'd talked to the Baiers in New Jersey. With one phone call he could talk to most of his family. His mother's brother is married to his father's sister, so they are essentially all one family. Because Bill's father is bedridden from a stroke, they all congregate at his parents' house for any holiday. It was nice to hear about all their news and messages of love. Bill also brought love from my brother, who lives near Dallas. I felt a little touch of Christmas reality as he delivered the messages.

Soon other Christmas visitors arrived. The pediatrician who was our family doctor stopped by with her husband. Bill had forewarned me that she was coming and that she was feeling responsible for my illness, since I had gone to her for a flu shot several weeks before I got sick. I didn't want her to feel guilty. We felt sure there wasn't any connection between my flu shot and Guillain-Barré.

When she saw me, she looked so devastated that I started crying. I understood what she was feeling, and I appreciated what it took for her to come here, especially on Christmas. I wanted so much to reassure her that this was not her fault. She didn't seem to notice Bill and the family. She just looked at me for a long moment, then turned away abruptly and left. I felt very sad. She was gone, still feeling responsible.

There was hardly time for me to compose myself before the arrival of Paul, the associate minister who worked with the youth at church. We knew him through his work with the girls' groups. I was touched by the generosity of his coming in on such a holiday. After initial pleasantries, his face became somber as he spoke of Nancy, a charter member of the church who was loved by all the congregation. "Nancy is in intensive care also, Sue. You might say a prayer for her." I heard Bill gasp.

Yes. But I had so many questions.

"She's had a heart attack. We don't know if she'll make it."

Nancy was a dear, thoughtful woman. I had just received a postcard from her a few days ago. It was unthinkable that she could be so ill now. The reality of it brought me up short. I wasn't the only person in the world in intensive care. And Paul wanted me to pray for her—that was something I could do for someone else. I wasn't totally useless.

Paul didn't stay long, but he helped me extend my world of concern beyond myself and the family. Now I had Nancy—and Cathy—to pray for. He had given me a new, positive sense of responsibility.

The nurse I had for the evening shift, three to eleven, was another Christmas gift. Carolyn was tall, nice looking, very articulate. I had never seen her before she announced herself with the nicest words. "I am at your disposal this evening. We'll do anything you want to do."

Shampoo!

"All right. Shampoo it will be," she said. "Just as soon as your company leaves for the night, we'll start."

Throughout the day, during quiet times, I looked around the unit. Many visitors came and went, but two patients never seemed to have any. How tragic to be left alone on Christmas. Had they no one, or were they just forgotten by people too busy celebrating the holiday? Perhaps they were too sick to notice. I almost hoped so.

Bill returned alone in the evening. I was so pleased with the nurses all day that I couldn't wait to tell him about them. I spelled to him that I had another good one this evening, and she was going to wash my hair. His smile showed relief.

Finally, Bill and I could shut out the rest of the world and have a few precious, peaceful minutes together—just the two of us, touching one another. At least I could share with him this tiny part of our traditional Christmas—these quiet, reflective moments at the end of the long, busy holiday. Silently I told him how much I loved him and thanked him for making my Christmas just a little more bearable by doing all those things I had asked for at home. What am I ever going to do for you, Bill, to repay you for all this?

That night, clean, fresh, and positioned comfortably, I settled in for a good night's sleep. Considering where I was, this was as good a day as I could have hoped for. This couldn't be a merry Christmas, but there would be other Christmases. I closed my eyes and pictured Bill and me at home together in front of the tree. Tonight, nothing else mattered. Through it all, I had Bill, Katherine, Elizabeth, Mother. I felt so loved. Certainly nothing could take that away from me.

10

During rounds on the day after Christmas, I watched hopefully for the three substitute nurses who had been so kind to me, but they were not there. Some of the regular staff did return from vacations, and I was relieved when I saw a few whom I knew. I hoped life would get back to normal again.

I was happily surprised that night when Peter was my respiratory therapist for the eleven-to-seven shift. That was unusual for Peter—he always worked days. Early in the shift he walked past my bed and looked up at the fluorescent light in the passageway over the clock.

"This light's still on," he said indignantly. "You've got to go to sleep. I'll go find a switch." Off he went in search of a switch, only to return looking very disturbed. "Sue, that light doesn't turn off!" How well I knew. But he was the first person who ever noticed or was concerned about that abominable light.

My nurse for the shift was new to intensive care. La Vonne knew I was supposed to be suctioned when I was repositioned. That was standard procedure. I'd watched it done so often, I could do it to myself if I were able to move. Several times, when I was heavily congested, my bed had been tilted, head down, to allow more of the phlegm to drain, but generally the procedure was done through the tracheotomy opening. The cap on the connection of the trach tube and respirator hose was removed, and saline solution was dropped into the trach to provide a medium for suctioning the lungs. Often the nostril opposite the NG tube was also suctioned. The respiratory therapist usually did all this, but it was time for the nurse to turn me, and Peter was not in ICU just then.

She called to Bruce, who was sitting in the nursing station. "I don't know how to suction," she said.

109

He looked up only briefly. "Oh, there's nothing to it."

"I'd be afraid to do it. I don't want to hurt her." She was standing by my bed; he remained seated at the desk.

"Oh, put in a couple of drops of saline and just do it." I could see she was frightened, and I couldn't understand why he wouldn't get out of his chair to show her. "There's nothing to it. You can't hurt her."

I felt her fear, and it was scary. She just barely went into the trach tube and tried to suction quickly. Nothing came. The drainage was still there when she left.

I was very happy to see Peter return, since my breathing was becoming difficult. I tried to tell him what happened, but my tears got in the way.

Our neighbor Julie's wedding was December 27. She had asked me to be a member of her house party. That was quite an honor, since I would have been the only older person in the party. I wanted so much to see her walk down the aisle, to help serve wedding cake or pour coffee at the reception. Bill, Katherine, and Elizabeth went to the ceremony, and Bill slipped away from the reception early to come to the hospital. He was getting much more observant about details he knew I enjoyed hearing. Elizabeth left the reception early too, he said, to finish packing for the ski trip, which began the next day.

Would she remember to take enough warm socks?

Early in the morning, Bill brought in Elizabeth to say good-bye. She had cut out the wedding portrait from the morning paper and held it so I could see as she described Julie's gown and mantilla. Julie looked lovely. That young man was very lucky to be getting such a sweet bride.

I asked her about the socks. Yes, she had plenty.

Be careful.

The sigh indicated her resignation to hearing those familiar words.

"Yes, Mother, I promise. I will be careful." Then she was off to meet the other skiers and catch the bus that would travel all day and night to the snowy slopes of New Mexico.

I was glad that she was able to go, but I was also concerned that she have a safe trip. They would be on the highways a long time, with all the holiday travelers and the bad weather that can blow up in West Texas and New Mexico.

The first time my respirator alarm sounded, I was terrified. I'd heard other patients' monitors go off and I knew it brought immediate attention, but I wasn't prepared for the proximity and the loudness of my own alarm. In the beginning, the alarms did bring immediate responses from the staff. But once they "knew" I was stabilized, they became less concerned, more casual.

Little things, such as a loose sensor, could trigger the alarm. Because of the difficulty of turning me, keeping the sensors attached was a constant problem. If the nurses were busy and felt sure I was all right, the alarm was a frustration to them—like a baby crying when its mother is dressing to go somewhere. A nurse would come to the cubicle, often obviously annoyed, and try to stick the sensor back on me. Usually that didn't work, and he or she would have to get a little kit and change the sticker, a bothersome task. In time, I became less frightened of the alarm, but I never overcame entirely the anxiety brought on by that piercing sound so close to my ears.

This night, when the respirator triggered the alarm, Bruce was my nurse. He was sitting at the desk in the nursing station—studying. He glanced over at me with that why-are-you-bothering-me-now look. Finally he set down his book and came to check the machine, found nothing wrong, and reset it. Then it happened again.

After several tries, he said, "You're fine. You're just going to have to live with that. I can't do anything about it." With that pronouncement, he returned to the desk and his studying. He never even tried to call anyone. While the alarm screamed in my ear, I knew the clamor had to be bothersome to him and everyone else in ICU, but no one did anything about it. I was Bruce's patient. After what seemed like an eternity, a relief therapist came running into my cubicle.

"How long has this alarm been sounding? Why didn't someone call me?" He was asking the wrong person.

Of course, I gave Bill the report on Bruce during his morning visit.

That night I had Louise again, and she force-fed me too much, too fast. I got a terrible case of gas. It was so unbearable that the charge nurse finally ordered that an antacid be poured down the tube to give me some relief. Then I was left in a heap again without my back-support pillow, and for two hours I tried to signal for help while I felt myself slowly falling over.

I was becoming terrified of Louise. Again I had to spell bad news to Bill in the morning.

Torture.

He looked startled, so I painstakingly spelled out what she had done.

Igno . . .

"Ignored," Bill repeated before we finished the word—some words I spelled frequently to him. Except for performing the required procedures, most of the nurses walked past me, never looking in so I could signal them. Please look at me, I pleaded silently. But it did no good. I tried to tell Bill that I must have someone with whom I could communicate.

"Sue, you know Dr. Lohmann said you can't have private nurses in ICU. It just isn't done."

Oh, please, Bill. Think of something. If only he realized how atrocious it was to be locked in this helpless, voiceless body.

"Sue, they can see you. You're right by the nurses' station. What more could you want?"

He still didn't understand. He had never even been hospitalized. How could I tell him that I want to be turned when I am sore and tired, not just when a clock or someone's mood indicates it's time. I want to be made comfortable. I want my mouth freshened and the perspiration washed off my face. I want to be looked at, talked to, seen as a human being. I want the same things any patient needs. But the others can speak; I can't. When you or someone else who communicates with me isn't here, right by my bed, I am shut out completely from the world and this ICU.

I could see the other patients using their call buttons, and the nurses responding to them. The call button is always clipped onto the pillow or bed after the sheets are changed. It is something nurses know is important—the patient needs to be able to call for help. But I was paralyzed; I couldn't move.

"You just have to try to get along with the staff, Sue." How can I try to get along with them when they won't even look at me?

Bill was wiping raindrops off his glasses as he came in for his evening visit. "It's been like this all day," he said, "just a steady drizzle."

Luzern.

He stopped wiping for a moment, then a broad smile crept across his face.

"Yes, like in Luzern. But you know Houston—rain slows traffic to a crawl." He put on his glasses, looking out of them at various angles to be sure he'd wiped off all the spots. Finally he settled into the chair next to the bed. "That *was* a good day, wasn't it?" I could almost see his mind drifting into a wistful reverie.

At the end of our first trip to Holland, we took a short Rhine River cruise and then traveled by bus to Luzern, Switzerland. The next day, we were scheduled to go up the mountain, but when we awoke, it was cloudy and rainy. Undaunted, we donned our raingear, protecting ourselves from head to toe, and took off on foot to see the city. We were delighted by the neat, charming houses, the bridges over the lake, the ducks and swans. We splashed through puddles, dashed in and out of shops, and played in the rain all day, like children.

The year we lived in Holland, we again visited Switzerland, and this time we did go up the mountains. The scenery was exquisite, breathtaking. But nothing could quite measure up to that funny, carefree day the two of us spent falling in love with Luzern.

I'd asked Bill repeatedly to figure out something that would work as a signal. I didn't know what it might be, but knowing how creative Bill is, I knew he could improvise something. And he was trying.

I was still able to twitch only my one leg muscle—nothing else, no matter how hard I tried. Bill watched me push that muscle again and again. Finally, one noon he was grinning broadly when he arrived carrying a package—jingle bells!

It was a foot-long strap of sleighbells, each bell a couple of inches in diameter. He laid the strap across my thigh, positioning it carefully so it wouldn't slide off.

"Now, move that muscle." I did. The strap fell off my leg and the bells jingled. It worked! A nurse passing by stopped to see what the sound was, and Bill was very pleased to explain to her, and the other staff, that this would be my call bell. He showed them exactly how to position it. Everyone agreed that it was a great idea—even the ones who never before considered me as human or conscious. I'm here, I wanted to tell them. I've always been here.

Now I had a way to attract attention. But I knew I had to save my signal for my most desperate needs. If I didn't, everyone would start to ignore the one-shot sound. I also realized that I must wait to call until someone was nearby who could spell with me. But I did feel more secure knowing that I finally had a "call bell."

Happily, Sandra was somewhat responsive to the bells, and she immediately learned to replace them correctly after answering the call. But too often, she heard the call and sent back the all-too-familiar "in a minute, Sue"—such as the night she was having coffee with a group of nurses in the station. That "in a minute" lasted thirty-five minutes. It seemed an eternity, not only because I needed straightening, but also because once I let the bells go, I had no way of calling for help in case of a real emergency.

If Sandra was tuned in, she could be great. But she seemed easily distracted. One night she had to change me, and before she was half-finished, Craig came by. Leaving me uncovered and ill-positioned, she went over to talk to him. Nurses are supposed to pull the curtain closed when they work on a patient, but she hadn't done it. So there I lay, totally exposed, for forty-five minutes. Occasionally she'd look back toward me and say, "I'll be right there, Sue." All I could do was lie there, watching the clock and crying. I felt stripped of all dignity. I have always been a very modest person, reserved and proper. This was ugly, and there was nothing I could do.

But when Sandra finished, she positioned me comfortably and carefully replaced the bell strip, completely unaware of how I had been humiliated.

A young patient was rushed into the unit. I'd seen him several times before in his wheelchair, visiting the staff. He always stopped by to talk to me, too. He'd been a long-term patient a while back and seemed to understand how I was feeling. It was obvious that the whole hospital loved him, and it was easy to see why. He was bright and pleasant to everyone. A nurse told me he'd been in a sledding accident and would be a paraplegic the rest of his life. Now he was placed on a tilt bed. Pneumonia again, they said; a chronic problem for him. I could see him just across the unit and one cubicle over from me. He was so young, only in his late teens, and he would have this problem the rest of his life. Here I was, unable to move and feeling sorry for myself, but I was lucky, knowing that someday I was going to walk again. He didn't have that hope.

I spent a great deal of time looking about the unit at the other patients. I saw them being brought in from surgery or the emergency room. They were all very sick and were hooked up immediately to monitors and often respirators. I saw doctors doing tracheotomies, and each time I felt a sense of apprehension. I felt sad for their worried families—and even worse for those who had no families to be with them. I wished I could move and talk so I could let those solitary ones know that I was pulling for them. They needed to have someone cheering them on, wanting them to get well. I knew now, more than ever before, how important that support was. But I was so useless, unable to help anyone.

Then I remembered Paul's asking me to pray for Nancy. *That* was something I could do for her and for the patients here—pray for them! Even if they were unaware of me, those who were all alone here would have someone pulling for them. I felt a bright, new sense of involvement, of worth.

One morning I watched the clock, very anxious for Bill to arrive. I always watched that clock for him, but this morning I had a treat for him, something good to report. Bill got out his book to take down the words. He always looked so dejected when I started right in as soon as he got there. By the third word, his face lit up.

Really good night. What a difference good nurses make.

He showed me the star he put in front of that message. Good news didn't come that often.

Weather forecasters were warning a cold night. I hoped Bill would remember to take in the plants. Everyone in the unit was talking about the weather, and I could feel the temperature in ICU cooling off. Suddenly I was startled to see Charles standing at the foot of my bed.

"It's cold out tonight." Surely he hadn't come to give me a weather report. I wished I could smile at him. Charles always brightened my cubicle when he was there. "It gets cold in here when the temperature goes down."

He remembered some socks that Bill had brought when he'd begun the tennis-shoe search, and he tugged them onto my feet. What a struggle!

"There. Those will keep your feet warm."

I'd already asked the nurse to cover me with a sheet, but Charles reached for a blanket and pulled it over the sheet. For the first time, a blanket felt good. After he had arranged the cover carefully, he stood for a moment and smiled. "There, that's better. Have a good night's sleep and I'll see you in the morning."

The next day Peter was cleaning my respirator. "I hear you had a visitor last night."

Yes.

Before I could say more, he said, "Charles slipped out from a dinner party and came over to the hospital because he was afraid you'd be cold and no one would notice." My heart filled with smiles. What a kind man.

Bill was pleased by Charles's thoughtfulness—and happy the socks finally had been put to use. His search for high-topped tennis shoes had proven futile. My feet were too difficult to fit and that style was impossible to find in this day of jogging shoes. He had been told he could abandon the mission after Charles had positioned a board at the foot of the bed to brace my feet and keep me from sliding out of the bed. My feet and I were grateful.

Bill had been trying for several days to call Dr. Lohmann to find out officially how I was doing. It was very hard to get through to him.

"I finally reached him today," Bill said.

News?

"Nothing new. He says you're doing fine." Before I could react, he continued. "I told him it was hard to catch him at the office, so he said I should call him at home." I could see that this made Bill feel good, and it would make things easier for him. This was more like the Dr. Lohmann I remembered. He had always made himself available when Mother needed him. If only he could see me as he used to when I was with Mother—as a person, not just an object to be reported on.

One day James noticed I was showing some lung power, but the slowness of other responses following my leg twitch taught me that I couldn't let myself get too excited about one little sign. The next day, the lungs did nothing on their own, but a day or two later, they again showed some indication of being able to work. Now I allowed myself more optimism.

Bill kept me posted on Katherine's New Year's Eve plans with the young man from Vanderbilt, and she came in herself, wondering what to wear. The previous year, we'd found a long, plaid taffeta skirt in red, green, and black. Perfect for the holidays, we had thought then. And it would be lovely with her green silk blouse. Katherine's eyes lighted up when I reminded her of the skirt. It was so good, so natural to be with her, happily anticipating her New Year's Eve.

Bill also brought news of friends. He had received many calls during the week, and he listed each one in his diary. His friend George from Virginia had taken his mother to Hawaii for Christmas, and now he was back, checking on me. During the trip, they'd sent me several postcards, beautiful scenes I recognized. I had gone to Hawaii after my first year of work at Shell. The maid of honor at my mother's wedding lived there, and she had always wanted me to come for a visit. So that's where I went for my first real vacation. And what a trip! My bedroom looked out over Diamond Head, and when the moon was out, I could see its form against the shimmering water. I was given the insiders' tour of Oahu, and Mother's friend and her husband arranged for the son of a friend to be my escort in the evenings. Her husband was in the import-export business and knew all the managers and maître d's of the best nightspots. Every place we went, we had front-row tables and the best of attention. I hadn't started dating Bill then, but I *had* met him. If I hadn't, I just might have looked into getting a job in Honolulu and staying there. It was a lovely fantasy world.

George remembered hearing me wish that Bill and I could go to Hawaii together, so he wrote in a card that this was a perfect time to get Bill—while he was feeling concerned about me—to promise a trip as soon as I was better. From the twinkle in Bill's eyes, I gathered that George had given him the same message on the phone. That would be fantastic. I would continue to think about that suggestion during my hospitalization!

Bill's best news was that Cathy was out of the hospital and Nancy was out of ICU. Good news was always welcome—anything that turned me away from concerns for myself.

The week after Christmas went quickly. Bill was more relaxed and had more time to stay with me. Also, he felt more comfortable making longer visits; the staff seemed relieved to have me taken care of for a while. Each time, Bill still took a handful of tissues and swabbed out my mouth and wiped off my face.

New Year's Eve sneaked up on me. I dreaded it. We had a tradition of getting together with Chickie and Hans for the evening. Tonight would be so lonely.

When Bill and I were married, Chickie had just met Hans. They were married soon after Katherine was born. From the beginning, the four of us enjoyed being together. None of us cared about big, noisy parties on New Year's Eve, so we got together at one of our homes, played bridge, and had a New Year's toast and midnight breakfast. It was a cherished tradition. One year, when their son developed an earache while we were there, Bill and Hans spent most of New Year's Eve running around Houston looking for an open drugstore to fill a prescription for ear drops. But still, we were together.

The tradition was not to be broken completely this year. Hans and Chickie brought Mrs. Flick—Oma—to visit me. I was very anxious to have her come, but distressed that she had to see me like this. I'd also dreaded the moment I would look into her warm, loving eyes again, knowing that she did not have long to live.

Now in her seventies, she was teaching herself English by watching American television programs. She had American grandchildren and was determined to communicate with them. Her letters to us, however, were still in Dutch, and Bill and Hans struggled through her intricate Dutch script to translate them. But we could always read the signature on her letters: *Oma*. And that is what she was to all of us. I had so looked forward to having her in my home, making it a wonderful visit for her, and now she had to come here to the hospital.

There was not much she needed to say. She took my hand and her smile was wonderful. In English she said, "Good to see you, Sue."

She brought a gift, a sachet. How typical. The Dutch bring gifts every time they visit anyone, and Oma was very generous—always bringing goodies for the children and something special for us.

Bill, Mother, and the girls had dinner with the Flicks earlier in the week and tried to prepare her for this moment, but that was impossible. I saw the sadness in her eyes, but I also saw the beauty of this woman. Tall and handsome, she had a certain glow about her that is hard to describe. After she left, several nurses stopped by my bed to ask, "Sue, who was that lovely woman?"

Chickie and Hans handled the conversation beautifully, interpreting my spelled greetings to Oma. And of course there was Chickie's kind gift to me—the dampened washcloth to clean off my face. As always, that was her first gesture when she arrived.

The visit was very special. I'd been worried about how Oma would handle this, but she was serene and loving. Her presence gave me a tremendous lift and a real lesson in courage.

The staff was anxious for New Year's Eve to be over. They dreaded this night because of all the accident cases that would be brought in. This was the only intensive care unit in the hospital, so we would get the results of any carnage in the area. I felt uneasy too—the staff would be too busy to do much for me.

As feared, there was a very bad accident. A mother and child were brought in. My heart wept for them. I prayed that they would make it. And I prayed for my own children—that they would be safe tonight.

The holidays were over now. I was glad. Although 1981 had begun unceremoniously, without my midnight kiss from Bill, I was thankful to see the new year arrive. It was a new beginning. Now we would lick this disease. This would be a very good year. I just knew it would.

11

New Year's morning I was upbeat. During the hectic night, Marie took time to give me one of her terrific backrubs. Because I couldn't lie on my stomach with the tracheostomy, and I didn't have the balance to remain unpropped on my side, my backrubs were a little unorthodox. I had to get them while I lay on my back. I loved the feeling of Marie's lotioned hands under me, kneading deeply up into my back. That made any night good.

Today, especially, I was thankful for the start of the new year. I was sure things would get better. I had to start improving if I were going to be well in two more months. Today I was certain it would happen.

Then Bill came in. One look at him and again I felt cheated—for both of us. We always watched the New Year's Day football games together, nibbling on snacks and taking down the holiday decorations. But today none of that would happen. Maybe I was fooling myself. Perhaps nothing else would start anew today either.

This was the last day of Bill's vacation, and what a dreadful one for him. In mid-December, he'd canceled his annual deer hunt—his one all-male activity of the year. Then his vacation was spoiled, too. He'd had none of the special good times of the holidays, just more work at home than ever before in his life. And all these days spent in this hospital. Dismal.

It was hard for us to think of anything to say. I reminded Bill that leftover turkey would make great sandwiches for his lunch back at the office. He nodded sadly and made a note in his book. Perhaps returning to the stimulus of his job would be good for him, a relief from the cloud that hung over the holidays. And there would be just one day, Friday, until the weekend—a good breaking-in time.

On Saturday, Mother came early and did my nails. The strain of this first Christmas without Daddy, and with me here in the hospital, showed all too clearly in her face. Not only was she worried about me, but I'm sure she missed the things we always did together. We've been extraordinarily close, I would say, for a mother and daughter. We are good friends. When I was growing up, we lived only thirty miles from downtown Houston, and we made that trip often. Mother and I would drive in, have our hair done, go to lunch, and perhaps do a little shopping. That was always a special treat.

When my brother and I were younger and we still lived in Houston, Mother was always home with us. Then Daddy left the insurance business and opened an auto dealership in the little town of Rosenberg. It was a family business, and Mother managed the office. But Fred and I never felt left alone. She handled it well. There were times, of course, when I had to go to the grocery store or fix dinner, and that probably annoyed me a bit at the time—even then, teenagers preferred to be free of household responsibilities. Mother also believed I should work with my brother at weeding the yard, and we had a large piece of land. In the hot summer, I found every possible excuse to get out of doing that.

Through the years, Mother had a number of illnesses that made it necessary for me to take care of her and the household. Perhaps there were times that it did interfere with what I wanted to do, but I was the other woman in the family. I realized early that this was my responsibility, something I needed to do. And Mother more than made it up to me during our special times together.

Now I found myself smiling as I remembered the time Mother had surgery during the summer following my sophomore year in college. I was in charge of the house while she was in the hospital recuperating. My good friend Mary Helen, who then lived in Galveston, came to spend a week with me, and she loved watching me keep house. With Mary Helen there, the job really wasn't work, because her companionship made it fun. Mary Helen and I still laugh about the permanent I gave her during that visit. I overdid the curl, and we giggled all the way to the beauty shop to get it all cut off before she went home. We still remember that week as great fun.

Now Mother needed some fun in her life. She looked tired and was quieter than usual. We will all be better with these holidays behind us, I thought.

After she left, I felt alone. No one came from physical therapy. Charles and Ginnie were both gone. I knew everyone was busy, especially with the overload from New Year's Eve, and ICU was short of staff. But knowing did not help. I needed some movement, and my body ached from not being turned often enough. This certainly was not shaping into a great new beginning.

ICU had a new head nurse. Mary Jean left word that she wanted to talk to Bill, so he prepared a long list of all the things he should speak to her about. He felt good about the meeting, sure that things would improve.

"She is very interested in you, Sue, and your case. I think she really understands." He was so confident. "She wants to do everything possible to make sure you get good care."

Within days it became obvious that nothing was going to change. Wasn't there anything anyone could do? Bill couldn't seem to accept my complaints.

"You have to give them time, Sue. Just give them time, and things will get better." Oh, Bill, how can I make you understand? I had only my eyes and a few spelled words to tell him what it was like to be treated roughly, to be seen as less than a person. Or not to be seen at all. These were intangibles, hard to convey, impossible for Bill to comprehend.

He did better with specifics. He reported to Dr. Lohmann that my ears were filling with wax. Sandra came in with the order to remove the wax. "Well, Sue, time to flush your ears." Hooray! What a relief it would be to have that done. She took a small container to the sink for water. Panic gripped me. I knew that, with the cool weather outside, the tap water from that sink would be frigid. I tried to signal her to test the water, but she never looked at my eyes. Into my ears she pumped what felt like freezing water. It stabbed my ears mercilessly. The pain brought tears down my cheeks, but Sandra never noticed.

Carefully she blotted the area around the ears. "There now, doesn't that feel better?" Her face showed much self-satisfaction, as if for a job well done. I told Bill to get the order for ear cleaning stopped. I couldn't take the chance that Sandra or anyone else would hurt me like that again.

I'd heard often about JoAnn. She was an assistant director of physical therapy, and Charles and Ginnie mentioned her name when they chatted together while working on me. Then I finally met her. She was as nice as I expected, a quiet young woman, kind and gentle. The first time she came in with Charles, she held my hand, working my fingers a little, but mostly just reassuring me. She spelled with me immediately.

One day she asked, "Is there anything you need, Sue?"

Ears clean. My hearing was becoming affected. I decided to take a chance that she'd ask a good nurse to do it.

"Well," she said with a grand smile, "I'll give it a try." And she did it perfectly with a small cotton swab. I was excited to find someone who cared enough to help me, even with things that were not her responsibility. "When you need it done again, just let me know."

By now I knew all of the procedures and the medications ordered for me—and when each was due. I diligently kept track of everything. Since becoming ill, my normal heartbeat had increased considerably, so Dr. Lohmann had prescribed Inderal to slow it somewhat. When my dosage was late even by fifteen minutes, I felt my heart begin pumping faster and my mind tensing. I admonished myself: This is not good for you, Sue. Relax. I knew the mind controlled much of the body, but my mind could not eliminate this racing heartbeat.

To help me remember the names of my medications, I used a word-association game. But I heard the name of this drug incorrectly, so I processed an association with what I thought I heard—"endure all." One morning, Carol was late with the dosage, and my heart began pounding. I signaled a nurse and spelled to her, but she couldn't figure out what I was saying. Finally she got Carol, and again I tried.

Carol laughed. "Oh, Sue, that's not how you spell it." I got my Inderal—and tried to think of a new word for my association. Carol was one of the few nurses who never became annoyed by my reminders.

The first week in January, Mother learned that an apartment she had signed up for in the fall was finally available. She needed to move, but she was overwhelmed with the idea of doing it without my help.

Bill and I were discussing the problem. There had to be some solution.

Ask Donna.

Bill considered the idea. "Well, Donna has called several times wondering what she could do to help. But isn't this too much to ask?"

She is interior decorator. Can suggest furniture arrangement.

I knew Bill hated asking for favors, but this one did seem logical to him. "I guess it won't hurt to ask."

It didn't hurt and Donna was happy to help. I also suggested that Mother call Bess and Sandy. Both were very willing, and together they set about getting Mother moved.

Donna began taking Mother out to shop for items she needed in the new apartment. They went often, each time picking out just one decorator item to tie her things in with their new environment. Mother carefully described to me a picture arrangement they were working on, and she brought in fabric samples for re-covering the dining-table chairs. These little shopping trips, often accompanied by lunch, gave her such a lift—just what she needed. For a few hours she was distracted from worrying about me.

By moving day, Bess and Sandy had all the smaller items packed and moved. I was so thankful that these friends not only were helping Mother but also filling some of the void that my illness had created.

One day a nurse stopped to ask if I knew someone named Marilyn.

Yes. Which?

"I think she belongs to a club with you. A literature club?"
Yes.

She smiled broadly. "Well, Marilyn just brought in coffee and cookies for all the nurses."

Marilyn was just an acquaintance—someone I saw at my literature club and occasionally at Bill's Rice alumni functions. She never contacted me directly, though I heard an aunt of hers had had Guillain-Barré. If her purpose was to make the nurses happy so they'd be nicer to me, it worked, and I was very grateful.

Vacation was almost over for Katherine, and Elizabeth was already back in school. I would miss their spontaneous visits. Katherine was getting ready to return to Nashville and was busy seeing former high school classmates before they all went their separate directions. Her first-semester grades came, and she made the dean's list. I was happy for her.

Elizabeth was effervescent about her ski trip. "I can't wait to go again!" Apparently the investment in ski clothes was not wasted. Besides, Katherine was planning a ski trip in the spring and would be borrowing some of them. That should please Bill.

Elizabeth was in the midst of school activities. Tonight it was the school board meeting. The Houston Independent School Board had voted to have a student from each high school sit in on board meetings—to become informed and involved. Elizabeth had been chosen from Lee High School. Students were encouraged to submit issues and questions through the board member from their area.

Since the girls would not be home until late tonight, I asked Bill for the first time to stay with me for a double shift of visiting hours. It had been a rough day, and I dreaded being alone all evening. Bless his heart, he did. He arrived at five-thirty and then waited to come back in during the eight o'clock visiting period. It was a lot to ask of him, but he did it without complaint.

From the beginning of my illness, I had recurring dreams that parts of my body could move. Then I'd wake up to the shattering reality. But on January 15, my head actually moved a little bit! I could consciously move it—not a lot, but it was movement. I had tested every muscle in my body, over and over, day after day, so I was startled with this sudden movement of my head. It was so exciting to have a response from something besides the muscle in my leg.

When Charles came in to do my range-of-motion therapy, he watched me show off my new skill.

"Wonderful!" he exclaimed. "Do it again." I obliged. Each time I did it, my head wobbled from one side to the other, rolling to a stop. Suddenly he dropped my foot.

"I know what you need!" He had that great big grin, and it looked like a light bulb had just gone off in his head. "Don't move. I'll be right back." Off he rushed, returning with a long, cylindrical pillow. He put it in a case and placed it under my head. It was wonderful. My head no longer wobbled or rolled to the side.

"There. Isn't that better?"

Yes! What a hallelujah day!

More frequently now, my lungs were giving the therapists some indication of beginning to work. Though I could not feel it happening, it was heartening to know. Bill made note of each forward step in my recovery. It fit the overall pattern, he told me, though mine seemed to be proceeding at a much slower pace than "normal." Bill was becoming very knowledgeable about Guillain-Barré, thanks to our friend Hans. Seeing Bill's frustration at not understanding my mysterious illness—and not getting satisfactory answers from anyone who did—Hans arranged for Bill to do research at the Baylor Medical School library. Bill spent every spare minute sleuthing out bits of information in medical books and journals—photocopying everything and giving copies to the therapists and the nursing staff in the hope that they were willing to learn. Now, finally, he could explain to me how Guillain-Barré attacks the sheathing of the neuromuscular system, destroying the nerve sheath and causing paralysis without necessarily destroying the feeling sensations. I could indeed ache, hurt, and know the pain of a poorly directed needle! It was such a relief to me that others could read the material and understand my plight. It was a relief, also, to know how my recovery would progress.

"You're coming back, Sue, just like it says!" Bill exclaimed.

Yes . . . yes.

"Some return quickly, others more slowly. The myelin sheath grows back at the rate of an inch a month." He paused for that to sink in. It did. With my height, it would take a long time to grow back all that tissue. "But you can twitch your leg and move your head a little, and your lungs are starting to work. You are getting better."

Getting better.

Bill clasped my hands firmly, and mentally I was also clutching his—we were like athletes, determined to win together. I might take longer to bounce back, but I *would* beat this disease and be back to a full life. I never doubted that I would make it—after all, Bill *told me* I would get well, but now I had written and physical proof, and I felt a new energy to fight.

The glow of such moments was transient. For all the moments that lifted our spirits, there were also the bad times, and my need to share them.

Louise hurts. Dumb.

I disliked burdening him with complaints, but I had to tell someone how frustrated and frightened I was. I got no sleep when Louise was my nurse. I was terrified of what she might do.

Marie took two hours to undo Sandra's mess.

My sentences became longer, perhaps in proportion to my frustration with the continuing foulups. Bill was also getting much faster at spelling with me. Words that I used more often became standards—even names were now familiar. Each word was preceded by the number of letters, which helped Bill.

Six blinks, then *S . . . a . . .*

"Sandra," he would say and simultaneously write in his book. "What did she do now?" He immediately recognized seven blinks and *Lo . . .* as Louise, or *Au . . .* as Aurilla. He knew that *Fol . . .* referred to a problem with my catheter.

Unfortunately, bad news often outweighed the good. And longer sentences meant more of it.

It remained agonizingly hard for me to deal with the limitations of our spelling system. Always just the barest facts. Never any remember-whens or small talk. I couldn't even tell Bill about the dream I had just before his morning visit. It was so real, the colors and smells so vivid. I wanted to tell him that I'd just dreamed we were back on the *France*, the ship on which we sailed home from Holland. In my dream the salt air was delectable and the music never stopped.

At the end of our Dutch exchange year, Tom and Sylvia invited us to sail back from Europe with them. Tom had been on sabbatical from his position at Rice University, and we'd met up with them twice on side trips—Switzerland for Christmas and London for Easter. When Sylvia first suggested sailing home, Bill laughed. All that time on a ship seemed silly to him, since his work demands a good deal of time on company boats, checking seismic equipment.

But Bill's co-workers in The Hague assured him that sailing was a wonderful way to return home. There's no jet lag, and it's so relaxing to have 4½ days when phones don't ring. We were convinced.

As we walked up the gangplank to board the *France*, my heart raced, and I couldn't believe it was real! Being on board with our friends made it all the more special. Their three children were fourteen, eight, and seven; ours were eleven and nine. They'd been together often enough by then to enjoy sharing the activities of the ship. We felt quite safe letting them wander the ship together, allowing the four adults time together, and giving Bill and me some very special time alone, just the two of us.

After dinner, we four often would wander into a little club where people gathered to avoid the big, formal ship parties. In my dream we were there, and Bill had promised me one last dance, but the musicians never stopped playing. On and on we danced, first in the club and then out onto the deck beneath the stars. The smell of the sea was intoxicating, and we kept on dancing. The children stood watching us, clapping as the music went faster and faster. And still we danced. Bill was saying, "I love you." Over and over he said it, all the while dancing faster and faster. I tried to answer. I tried to say, "I love you, too." But we were dancing too fast. I had no breath.

"I love you, Sue."

I was trying so hard, but I couldn't say anything. Even when I opened my eyes and saw Bill bending over me, I couldn't say the words. There was no breath. Oh, Bill, I want to tell you once more how much I love you. The single tear that dropped from his eye to my cheek, and the tenderness of his voice, told me he knew.

Katherine was leaving for Nashville on January 11. When she visited me earlier, I sensed her anxiety about going through "rush" to join a sorority. I wanted to talk to her once more before she left, to give her a little moral support. Bill promised to bring her to the hospital on their way to the airport. He warned me that they would be in a hurry, but he would time it so I'd have a half hour to spell my best motherly pep talk to her.

Marie, bless her heart, was my nurse that morning. She was such a good nurse, and on this day she had time to give me a thorough bath. She wanted it to be a special treat. However, she fell behind schedule, and the doors to ICU were closed to all visitors until my bath was finished. As she worked, I watched the clock. We were running late for Katherine and Bill. I tried to spell to Marie to finish up and let them in, but she kept right on talking and primping me. There was nothing I could do. She used up the entire half hour I so desperately wanted with Katherine.

When the door opened for visitors, Katherine and Bill rushed in and kissed me. "No time to talk," Bill said. "We have a plane to catch." With only a few words and another kiss, they were gone.

It wasn't Marie's fault. Without speech, I had no way to communicate with her. She was determined to give me a little of the special attention she knew I wanted and needed. But now Katherine was gone, and I had no time even to remind her that I loved her.

Two weeks later, rush week was well underway, and I waited for news from Katherine. My week was not going well—my temperature was up again—and I grew concerned for Katherine, too. I was beginning to suspect that no news from her was bad news. Finally, when my temperature returned to normal, Bill gave me the word: Katherine did not pledge. I knew how disappointed she must be, and I hurt for her. If only I could have talked to her before she left. She still would have had to bear the disappointment of not getting something she wanted, but maybe I could have made it a little easier for her to face. And now. . . . I wanted to talk to her, to write to her, to tell her how much I loved her and how little this mattered. And how proud we were of her. Oh, why this illness? I cried for two days. Dear God, please take care of her, of all my family. I wanted to ask Him to take care of me, too, but that was harder. The people at church would take care of that for me.

Tears in ears, I spelled.

Bill studied me after realizing that this was all of the message. His shoulders slumped when he understood. I'd been crying, and the tears were accumulated in pools in my ears. Tenderly he twirled cotton swabs to soak them up. I didn't need to tell him why I had been crying. He wiped away more than tears.

Days were interminable, and evenings were even worse. After Bill left at six, time was empty, but I didn't want him to stay at the hospital any later. Darkness comes early in January, and I didn't want Elizabeth to go home to an empty house. That was unthinkable to me. In ICU, the pace of evening visitors slowed in January. Dark hospital parking lots are a deterrent. Most of those who still came faithfully obeyed the posted fifteen-minute visiting notice. Only Bill, Mother, and a few close friends stretched their time. With increasing therapy, the lengthy feedings, and Bill's and Mother's visits, the days were a little less lonely—even if the increased activity was frustratingly tiresome. But the evenings alone were terrible. Television would have helped, but it interfered with the hospital equipment in ICU and was not allowed.

I was astonished the day Bill brought in a tiny, battery-operated TV set. Dr. Lohmann finally told him that yes, this was a serious case, and I would be here for a while. So Bill persuaded the staff to allow this little five-inch set. I was so excited. I thought I might even shout. After removing it from the box and inserting the batteries, he adjusted the tuning and focusing—and finally we had a picture. It was wonderful!

After some experimentation, Bill positioned the set on the crank-up table, which he rolled to the foot of the bed. I was very excited, but I also realized I would have another responsibility—keeping track of my television set. That table was used beside the bed during the day for small equipment and for my bath water. I must make sure that no one knocks my television off the table or spills water on it. No sooner had I thought about that than Bill repeated my thoughts. Had we lived together that long?

Yes. Will watch.

We tried to remember which of my favorite programs were on this evening. Whatever channel I selected had to remain on the whole evening. By the end of his visiting time, Bill had it set for me. Now there was something to look at besides that yellow wall and the clock. Dear, thoughtful Bill. How I want to throw my arms around you and whisper thank you. I hoped he knew my tears were from happiness and gratitude. His smile said he did. He turned quickly and left, reaching for his handkerchief from a hip pocket.

Now Bill had to remember disposable batteries for the television every other day, rechargeable batteries for the radio every day, and the weekly issue of *TV Guide* to help me select my station for the night.

As my lungs increased their ability to assist the respirator a little, the therapists began changing the setting of the machine for brief periods—to make the lungs work harder. The new setting, which they referred to as IMV, was very frightening, especially when it was done by someone who was not good with me, or if I was left alone. On the new setting, the machine seemed to pause, trying to force me to breathe. But I could not control my lungs to make them inhale. If I didn't breathe sufficiently for a certain number of seconds—which seemed like an eternity—the machine would supply me with another few breaths and then pause again. It was exhausting to struggle with the irregular pattern of breathing, and coping with the fear left me completely drained.

James's bright face was always a welcome sight when he came to work with me. At least when he was there and I had to face these dreadful episodes with the respirator, there was a reassuring hand holding mine—and someone who thought to reward me occasionally by returning the respirator to the normal setting for a few minutes so I could rest.

One evening I learned another of his talents. My nurse turned me and tried to position me, without success. James walked by and she called to him. "I can't get Sue settled right. Will you help me?"

Without a moment's hesitation, he took over. He knew exactly how to place the pillows. With little effort, he had me positioned perfectly. When he returned later to suction me, I learned he was also a nurse. Later the nurse tried again to position me and gave up, leaving me in a heap. An hour later, James checked the respirator and saw the mess I was in. Again, with ease, he settled me, relaxed and comfortable, for sleep.

After that, whenever I had an evening nurse who was unable to turn me comfortably, I'd tell Bill, *Ask James fix me*. And James would watch me the rest of the evening, repositioning me whenever I needed it. I wished that I could speak to him, but perhaps there was nothing to say. Certainly no mere words could tell him what his caring meant to me. I could relax when he finally finished, smiled, patted me on the leg, and said, "There! See you tomorrow, Sue."

Vickie was bubbling these days when she was my nurse. I sensed something special was happening. "Sue, I have to tell *someone*. I'm going to tell you, but not anyone else. They'll spread it all over the hospital, and I don't want everyone to know yet." She looked around for eavesdroppers. "Sue, I'm pregnant."

So happy.

With frequent looks over her shoulder, she told me about going to the doctor and breaking the news to her husband.

As soon as Bill came, I signaled him that I had a message. He reached for his book and wrote down the letters.

Vickie pregnant. Secret.

Bill Baier couldn't let that slip by unnoticed. When Vickie came in to turn me at noon, he said very quietly, "I understand we have some news, Vickie." She looked at his grin for a moment, smiling herself, and then turned to me, hands on hips.

"I told you not to tell anybody. A fine thing. I can't even trust you, Sue."

Secret. Promise.

And I kept my promise. I was so happy for her. She would be a wonderful mother.

My daily routine had its bright moments when staff shared their lives with me. Carol's stories of her cats were now usual whenever she had me. She knew how much I missed our Tiffany, and I loved her feline tales. Charles was going to try a new diet—after next weekend's big dinner party.

Others talked about their home lives and families. Luana was a petite, young Indonesian woman who was married to a Texan. Now they had a baby, and this, she announced, made them all true Texans. Luana only worked two days a week, but it was always two shifts together. I could never understand how she handled those long days. But whenever she had me, I looked forward to her talk of her husband and baby—and to fine nursing care.

Joan, also an Indonesian, was almost late for work the day it snowed in the northern suburbs of Houston. Everyone teased her because she had taken her little girl to see snow. But I understood perfectly. When Katherine was six months old, we took her to New Jersey for the holidays. To my delight, it snowed on Christmas! Fortunately, Katherine was prepared for the cold weather, thanks to Nana's insistence that I order a bunting for her. Such apparel was not common in Houston. I bundled Katherine in her new pink bunting and took her out in the blizzard to see her first snow. Bill dutifully recorded this big event with our camera. But I was the only one who seemed thrilled. Katherine didn't understand snow, and part of the family couldn't come for dinner because of bad roads. I felt bad about that, but still I loved this White Christmas. Later in the day, Bill and I went for a long walk. It was beautiful, and it's now a cherished memory. I completely understood Joan's taking her little girl to see snow. I wished I could have gone with her.

At home, Bill was busy sending thank-you notes for all the help, the food, and the gifts. And little by little, he was removing and putting away the Christmas decorations. Katherine was gone, and Elizabeth was busy with school, so her help was sporadic. Poor Bill. There was no end to his lists of chores.

People from church continued to bring prepared dinners every few days. They were organized with a schedule now. In between, there were meals delivered and dinner invitations from friends—and plenty of leftovers. Still, Bill had his job, three trips a day to the hospital, all the household and financial responsibilities—even his own lunch to pack every day. He looked so tired that it began to concern me. Yet I continued to add to his burden with my problems about forgotten procedures, my complaints about the staff, and my messages to the doctors. I had no one else to act as my voice. Please forgive me, Bill, for being such a burden.

One day a man in a jogging suit appeared in ICU. His attire was a wonderful contrast to the staff uniforms and the no-nonsense appearance of the visitors. The nurses were obviously pleased to see him and immediately escorted him over to my bed. He exuded the smell of fresh air. It turned out that he was a former ICU patient who hovered near death for some weeks as the result of an automobile accident.

"Now," Marie instructed him, "you tell Sue that we got you up and out of here, and we're going to do the same for her." He was so jovial and reassuring that he truly lifted my spirits.

Some patients, however, did not make it in ICU.

It was never a secret what was happening. A patient's monitor triggered the alarm, and all the staff went running. "Code blue" echoed through the unit. A nurse rushed by, pushing the crash cart loaded with lifesaving equipment.

Sometimes their mission was successful, but when it wasn't, I'd hear the long, flat tone that meant they'd lost the battle. Slowly, everyone would disperse—their expressions showing the sadness of loss. I, too, was sad. I wanted all of us patients to walk out that door to a full life after these dreadful days.

After a patient died, the body had to be removed. When the men came for the removal, a nurse rushed around the unit and pulled the curtains across all the cubicles. It was a routine gesture, an effort to spare the other patients. But because I had no reliable call button, the terror of having that curtain close me off from everyone was sheer torture. My heart would race, regardless of when I'd had my last medication. Terrifying isolation would swirl around me, and I was sure I was being swallowed. Minutes were interminable. Eternity was now.

Although this situation occurred an average of once a week, I never conquered the fear. I knew no relief from it until the day James was standing just beyond the foot of the bed as the curtain was drawn. Apparently he caught a glimpse of my desperate look of anxiety, and in he came to inspect the machinery he'd just checked a half hour earlier. He stayed until the curtain was opened again. Dear James, thank you.

From then on, whenever he was available to stay with me, I never had to face that horror alone. Immediately James would appear, usually carrying a stack of charts. He'd sit on a stool near the edge of my cubicle, scribbling and shuffling. Sometimes he'd smile and thank me for allowing him to use my stool for his charting. But he was there, soothing me with his presence.

Flu was rampant in the hospital. Staff members were out, and I heard nurses talking about the large number of patients admitted with this bad virus. If there was one thing I did not need now, it was the flu! Kay obviously was coming down with it, but she was so conscientious she stayed on. I prayed I would not catch her virus.

A few nights earlier, Kay had noticed that the respirator showed signs of leaking. Finally, it had to be replaced. She went for a new one, but it had to be serviced before startup. To keep me breathing, Sandra pumped air into my lungs with the Ambu-bag, rather like a bellows. For two hours she stood next to me, bagging me by hand with a regular pattern of breathing. We could both watch Kay, working as fast as she could on the new respirator while fighting flu symptoms. All the while, Sandra and Kay talked to me and spelled. Sandra must have been getting terribly tired, but she never missed a beat. And all through it, she kept reassuring me. I was completely relaxed with her. It amazed me that she could be so dreadful at times, and could show such patient endurance at other times. I was enormously grateful to Sandra and Kay for what they were doing, but especially for two hours of uninterrupted companionship.

Kay was out sick the next few nights, but I never got the flu.

January 18: the day before Bill's birthday. There was nothing I could do to make the day special for my husband. I was afraid he might forget—or, worse, that Elizabeth might.

Tell Elizabeth your birthday tomorrow.

He grinned. "Don't worry, Sue. She remembered. There have been broad hints."

The next morning, before I could spell Happy Birthday, he said, "The kitchen is such a mess. You wouldn't believe!" I didn't believe—or understand.

"Elizabeth made strawberry crêpes this morning." Oh, thank you, Elizabeth! Bill loves strawberry crêpes—the kind filled with cream cheese and topped with sour cream and strawberries. Whenever we go to a pancake restaurant, that's what he orders. And to think I was afraid Elizabeth would forget what day it was! She had to leave for school by seven, but she'd gotten up and done that for her father's breakfast. No wonder she didn't have time to clean up the kitchen! I was touched that she'd made such an effort, all on her own.

He was still shaking his head, practical old Bill. "You should just see the kitchen." Inside I grinned from ear to ear, but all Bill could see were the happy tears that squeezed from my eyes as I spelled. *Happy birthday.* Next year, dear Bill, I'll make sure you have a really happy birthday. There will be crêpes for breakfast, your favorite sauerbraten for dinner, and a gathering of the whole family. And laughter and teasing and fun—and a clean kitchen!

Bess removed a letter from her purse and unfolded it. "Lissy wanted me to read this to you," she said. Lissy was her daughter, between Katherine and Elizabeth in age, and our two families had been close since the girls were in junior high school.

> Dear Mrs. Baier,
> I just thought you might like a little report on the goings-on around Lee. . . .

How dear of her. Of course, I always wanted to know everything about Lee High School. She gave Elizabeth rave reviews on her participation at school and told about a very special conversation she'd had with Katherine. She even teased me that I now had the "Mo Ranch Revenge"—a reference to the previous summer, when Lissy spent a weekend with us at our church's family camp, Mo Ranch. Unfortunately, a terrible stomach virus hit and felled most of the hundred-plus campers one by one. I didn't want any of us to get sick, but I was especially concerned about my responsibility for Lissy. All the teenage girls slept in one large dorm, away from the parents. I told Elizabeth and Katherine that I wanted to know right away if they or Lissy got sick. In the middle of the night, one of the campers marched across the campground in the dark to get me. "Mrs. Baier, you wanted to know if Lissy got sick. Well, she is." By the time I got to the dorm, Elizabeth and Katherine also were sick. It was a long, busy night with all three girls. I was one of the few people there who wasn't attacked by the virus. But I did get such a virus a few days before Thanksgiving—and that may have triggered this awful disease.

. . . I always knew that you couldn't escape the Mo Ranch Revenge forever.

> I love you,
> Lissy

It was a sweet letter, and I was touched that she'd thought to write me. When Bess finished reading, she refolded the letter, put it back in her purse, told me a few bits of news, and was gone. I tried to signal her—I wanted that letter. It was a treasure.

First thing next morning, I spelled the assignment to Bill, who retrieved the letter for me.

"January 20: Clean. Put out tree."
                                          —from Bill's diary

When the Iranians first took over the American Embassy in Teheran, I felt concern for the hostages and their families. The news was always headlined in Houston, because the mother of one of the captives lived here. But in ICU, I felt a special kinship for the hostages. I, too, felt like a prisoner—a captive of a disease, lingering at the mercy of so many strangers who now controlled my life.

As efforts to negotiate the hostages' freedom escalated, I became increasingly depressed. I couldn't understand why. I wanted them to be free, but who was negotiating for my freedom? When the release appeared imminent, I watched televised reports with a passion. Yellow ribbons were hung from trees all over the country to prepare for the welcome home. Yet, I was filled with apprehension. Would they really be set free or would something happen at the last minute to undo all the planning, to shatter all the hopes? I wanted them to make it.

When it happened, when I saw them on my TV set, coming off the plane in Germany, I was overcome with envy. I watched scenes of the homecoming of the Houston man, his mother's tears of joy, and all the yellow ribbons hung throughout the city. I was jealous. I, too, wanted to be free. But I was still the hostage.

Each evening when Bill read the TV listings to me, I wanted to hear everything, even the schedule for the old-movie channels. One night I chose *Bedtime for Bonzo*. What fun it would be to see our newly inaugurated president back in his early acting days. After a miserable day, a comedy would be welcome relief. I was having a pleasant time all by myself—until fifteen minutes before the end of the movie. A nurse came by and shut it off. "Sleep time," she proclaimed. She had never even looked at me. This was such a little thing to be upset about, I told myself, but it was one more of the many thoughtless acts heaped upon me every day. I had absolutely no control over any aspect of my life.

I kept remembering Daddy and his days in the nursing home. Had he known that his life was out of his control? I remembered the faces of other elderly men and women at that home—one of the good homes. Many of them still had a spark of awareness in their eyes. Did anyone ever look into those eyes and try to see what was behind them?

I looked around the unit at the others, who seemed to be asleep. Were they? Had they also been informed summarily that it was "sleep time," so they gave up and went to sleep, or perhaps pretended? This was only one small hospital. How many more of us were there in other hospitals who wanted to shout that we were not yet ready for sleep?

I wished I could be a little more sure that Daddy didn't know what was happening in the world that surrounded him at the nursing home.

A new player entered my game. I heard the nurses call him Dr. Birmingham, and James said he was an anesthesiologist. I couldn't imagine why an anesthesiologist was involved in my case. But he seemed to live in ICU and gradually began stopping by my bed, looking at my chart, and asking the nurses questions about me.

He was a large, imposing man, partially bald, with a fierce temper that was often the topic of conversation in the unit. He always had a nurse with him as he made his way around the

ICU, but those who didn't have to be with him scooted out
sight whenever he approached, because so often he castigat
anyone at hand. I tried to understand how he was connected to
my case, especially when he began giving orders to the staff
concerning my care. Dr. Lohmann had never mentioned him as
a consultant. No one ever explained how he got authority over
my care—specifically, over the setting of my respirator. But even
Bill was recognizing him as one of my doctors.

"Dr. Birmingham says you're afraid of the machine," Bill
reported.

*Tell him not afraid of machine, but of help who don't know
how to work it.* Dr. Birmingham wasn't there when a nurse tried
to "adjust" my life support and fouled it up.

Dr. Birmingham came to my bed several days later. He said
nothing about my message, but he ordered James to turn the
respirator to a higher IMV setting, with longer gaps to force my
lungs to work even harder. It was terribly uncomfortable and
frightening. He was trying to make my lungs do more than they
were capable of doing.

My eyes pleaded with James, and he looked at Dr. Birmingham, who didn't seem to notice my fears. "She should be
ready for this. Keep it going." Terror was mounting.

Within minutes, he realized I wasn't ready. "She's not taking
enough; set it back," he said, seeming annoyed. My heart raced.
"She should be ready by now, but I guess we'll have to ease her
off more slowly." From now on, he ordered, the setting would be
adjusted gradually every three or four days.

Nothing seemed to be progressing fast enough, or on any
predictable schedule. At times I felt as if some people thought I
wasn't trying hard enough. It wasn't my fault, honestly. I was
trying. Oh, I was trying.

*"January 25: Birmingham cries. Says Sue may never breathe on
her own again."*
—*from Bill's diary*

Something was wrong, I didn't know what, but I was scared. I was having trouble breathing. I was not getting enough air. Often I'd been anxious when the respirator's IMV setting was increased, but I was familiar with that sensation. Something different was happening to me—and, of all nights, it was when Aurilla was my nurse and Bruce was in charge of the shift. Perspiration poured off me. Frantically, I waited for Bill to come; he had to find out what was wrong.

Bill took one look at me and knew we had a problem. He turned quickly toward the station. "Who's Sue's nurse?" Aurilla strolled over to the cubicle.

"Something is wrong with her. Is the respirator working properly?"

Aurilla was unimpressed. "I'm sure it's fine. She just gets upset when it's on IMV."

"It's more than that this time."

Without responding, Aurilla took my pulse and then my blood pressure.

"She's just fine. Everything is normal," she reported.

"How normal?"

"Her pulse is sixty-two. That's normal."

"Not for Sue it isn't normal!" After all this time, Aurilla and many of the other nurses still did not seem to remember that my heartbeat always was much faster on the respirator. That is why they gave me the Inderal. "Sue's normal is 112! Something is wrong. Turn the machine back to the regular setting," Bill was ordering. "Get it off the IMV until we find out what's wrong."

Aurilla said, "You'll have to talk to Bruce about that. He's the charge nurse tonight."

Bruce never got up from his desk, never came over to check my pulse or the respirator. He just sat there and announced that he couldn't change the setting. "I have Dr. Birmingham's orders not to move the dial."

"But there's something wrong. You have to change it." Bill was being polite but forceful.

"Without a doctor's order, I can't touch it."

Bill's frustration was soaring, as was my panic. Suddenly he spotted Dr. Muenkel walking into ICU. With noticeable relief, Bill called to him. Dr. Muenkel ordered the setting changed immediately. "Now, let's get her suctioned," he said. And to everyone's amazement, out came a huge mucus plug. What a relief! Now I could breathe comfortably again, and my heart-beat went back to normal, my normal.

As Bill was leaving for the night, he saw Dr. Birmingham at the nursing station. Obviously Bruce had told him what had happened. When Bill approached them, Dr. Birmingham put his arm around Bruce's shoulder and, with a *very* nice smile, said, "Bruce is one of our finest people, you know." Bill asked the doctor about his orders, and again he smiled. "Well, of course, if things had really gotten bad, Bruce would have changed the setting."

Next morning, when Bill told me about the conversation, I was incredulous. Those two were delicately shifting the blame so nobody would be found guilty of a mistake! That morning Mary Jean talked with all the ICU staff, instructing them about the suctioning and telling them that this should never have been allowed to happen. Finally!

I had become frightened whenever I saw Dr. Birmingham in ICU, and I had good reason for fear two days later when he announced that he needed to change the tracheostomy appara-tus. This meant that I would be off the respirator while he made the change. By now, the outer facing of the trach tube adhered to my skin. The pain was excruciating as Dr. Birmingham tore the tube away from my neck. Was he completely devoid of feelings, of awareness that I could feel? It seemed an eternity that I was off the respirator. The sound of my heart pounding with fear echoed in my head. My terror was deafening. I tried to watch what he was doing, but he was so near and overpowering that I closed my eyes to remove him. That was my only defense.

It was becoming quite obvious that I would not be well in the promised three months.

My first time off the respirator was a red-letter day, although I wasn't entirely aware of what was happening until it was over.

Harriet and Kay came to my bedside, looking very conspiratorial.

"This is it, Sue Baier," Kay said. "Today you are going to try something new and exciting! We're going to try you on pure oxygen."

Before I could spell my questions, Kay read them in my eyes.

"You're not to worry. We're just going to try this for two minutes, and Harriet and I will be right here with you. If you feel any discomfort . . ." Already I was uncomfortable about this unknown. Nervous perspiration was beading up all over my face. ". . . you just blink twice. We'll switch you right back."

Yes. Only my faith in Kay and Harriet, who had become my friends, made me tell them it was all right. Kay hooked a plastic tube to the oxygen outlet on the wall.

"All right, Sue," Kay said. "Are you ready?"

Yes. We could try. Here we go. She switched the tubes at my trach. My eyes were fixed on Kay.

I couldn't feel anything happening. "You're doing fine, Sue. Keep on. Think breathing." I tried to imagine myself taking a breath, but I felt nothing. Still, Kay was cheering me on with such enthusiasm.

"Look," Harriet said, "she's taking some." A minute and a half.

"Keep on, Sue. You're breathing. Just try twenty seconds more." I'll try, Kay. I don't feel like I'm breathing, but I'll keep trying.

"You made it!" They both cheered as Kay changed the connection. "You made it."

"Two minutes," Kay said, "is a start, Sue. And you did it!"

Their excitement was infectious. I had made a major step forward! Finally!

That evening, when Bill visited me, there were no complaints. Before he left, I spelled one word: *hug.*

There were tears in Bill's eyes as he reached carefully around all the tubes and sensors and held me in his embrace. For a brief moment our closeness allowed us to escape the horrors of this place.

12

"Look at your December bill." Bill was holding up a bale of computer paper, a stack at least 1½ inches thick. "I just wanted to show it to you," he said, waving it in the air aimlessly. He was struggling with his bewilderment.

I was shocked. He read random items aloud, but this was all too much for my mind to comprehend. Yet I should have guessed. Every time the staff used anything on me, they took the sticker off the item and posted it on the wall chart, which was removed at the end of each shift. I knew hospital bills included charges for patient kits—the toothbrush, water pitcher, and tissues—plus the per-day charges. And if they used a special piece of equipment, such as a heating pad, they charged extra for that. But here it was. Every single swab, every single anything was listed line by line! I couldn't believe they were charging per piece. Whenever I was suctioned, the therapists used a little plastic box into which they poured distilled water to dip the tube for suctioning. For every time this was done, there was a charge for that little box and the distilled water—not to mention the charge for the therapist's visit.

Strangely, of all the charges posted, it was the lemon swabs that bothered us most. Bill held one up and said, "Do you know how much this one swab costs? Sixty cents." That was incredible! Imagine this little item costing sixty cents when I could go out to a store and buy a whole box of them for $1.29. It was good Bill was still bringing in my tissues. Our large boxes were less expensive than the hospital's tiny ones.

This was just the first month's bill. Bill assured me that we had good insurance, so I needn't worry, yet both of us were disturbed. Every time I saw a sticker plastered up on the wall chart, I thought about the next month's bill.

I was lying on my side facing the machine. Aurilla had just turned and suctioned me. My eyes focused on the alarm switch. It was off! That can't be. My alarm can't be turned off! What if something happens? From the corner of my eye, I looked out into the unit. No one. Please, someone, my alarm is off. Four o'clock. Bill won't come for two hours. James, where are you? When I was suctioned, the respirator setting had to be changed. To keep the alarm from sounding during the procedure, Aurilla turned it off until the machine was reset. But she had forgotten to switch the alarm back on.

My heart was racing. Fear churned my stomach. If something goes wrong, no one will know. The bell won't go off to warn the staff. Is the machine working now? Is it set right?

I never could feel my breathing—not since I was put on the respirator. I tried to look down to see if my lungs were expanding, but I was on my side, and my gown was puffed away from my body. But I *had* to be breathing. Otherwise Bill said I would pass out.

I stared at the respirator. It sounded right, the same as it always did, but was it? And what if it stopped? What could I do? I had no way to call for help. Fear screamed in waves of nausea. Perspiration turned clammy.

The first time I caught movement in my peripheral vision, I tipped the sleighbells. The nurse did not notice. Now I had no call button. My eyes flashed a signal to anyone who passed my cubicle, but no one saw. For over an hour I lay waiting in dread. Finally James came in.

Alarm!

As he flipped the switch to the on position, tears poured from my eyes. I didn't dare cry before now. I had to see and be ready to signal. James gently wiped away the tears and perspiration. "It's all right now, Sue," he said. "I'll try to watch more closely after this." The intensity of his voice told me I could believe him. But what was I to do when James wasn't on duty?

Above the sibilance of the respirator I heard the staccato of James's voice at the nursing station. Perhaps he could do something. Please listen to him, please listen and remember.

Most of the good nurses were part-timers. Sometimes Bonnie came only one day a week. Luana came twice a week. Carol usually worked four days one week and then only a weekend the next. Scheduling seemed haphazard. They all seemed to come and go without any continuity or certainty. Even those who were good had to relearn what was happening with me after several days off. At times several good nurses worked the same shift, and I would get one of them. But then days passed without my having a nurse who cared enough, or had time, to communicate with me.

And, of course, there were full-time nurses—Bruce, Aurilla, Phil. Always there. Especially Aurilla.

As Charles gave me range of motion one afternoon, I shot a look in the direction of Aurilla.

"Ah, you have her again." His sigh spoke volumes of understanding. "I'm sorry, Sue. I tried. I told them how you feel about her. There's nothing more I can do."

Even James tried to persuade Mary Jean, the head nurse, to keep Aurilla away from me. It didn't work. "But don't worry. I'll watch you evenings when she's on." Thank you, James, for being my security blanket.

One Sunday morning I was startled to see Aurilla making rounds. She never worked days. I felt a dull thud in my stomach, knowing I'd surely have her again.

Things had been chaotic in the unit all night, with several "codes" and two other critical patients. Before Bill arrived, Phil, who was in charge this shift, came over to my bed. "Sue, I'm going to apologize now for giving Aurilla to you," he said, "but we can't risk giving her to somebody who's really sick."

It was incredible. I'd known all along how bad she was, but nobody—not even Bill—seemed to believe me. And now Phil was finally admitting it. I wanted to plead, Why is she here? If only Bill were here to listen to the truth.

Patiently Bill wrote the words in his diary and nodded his head, as he did routinely. But did he comprehend? Did he believe? Surely he didn't think I was imagining this conversation with Phil. "But what can we do, Sue? Dr. Lohmann says you're getting good care. We don't want to make trouble."

My brother came in from Dallas to help with Mother's move. Fred would supervise the movers, hang pictures and mirrors, and take care of other matters. He and Mother came to the hospital the night before moving day. It had been a long time since our last visit, so I was delighted to see him. He'd called Bill several times to inquire about me, but I'd felt a twinge of sadness that he hadn't come to visit me before. Now I could see how much the sight of my condition was affecting him. Perhaps he had known what he was afraid to face. Tears poured down his cheeks. I had never before seen my brother cry. He was always the strong brother, even though he is three years younger. Now we were both older—so much older tonight. He was barely able to speak to me, but he promised to come back after the move was completed. By then, I was sure, he'd be more comfortable with how I looked and would be able to talk with me as we used to do. Funny how just seeing him brought back so many memories of our childhood years.

Fred and I played well together as youngsters. Only once do I remember a real blowup between us. Fred was a tease, as brothers can be. I don't remember what he was doing that time, but he infuriated me, so I picked up the red fire truck he had gotten for Christmas and threw it down and broke it. Even now, years later, he loves to tell that tale on me, and it still embarrasses me. I just didn't do things like that!

After Fred and Mother left the hospital, they stopped at a cafeteria to have dinner, and during the night they both became extremely ill from food poisoning. But they had to continue with the move the next morning. Mother said poor Fred did well to keep going, but he was too exhausted to come back to see me. Besides, he had the long trip home ahead of him. I was very disappointed that I couldn't see my brother before he left. I would gladly have endured the fire-truck story again!

In spite of being exhausted herself, Mother visited me and chatted pleasantly about what Fred had said and about all the help my friends had given her. I tried not to let my eyes show how sad and useless I felt. I was the one who should have been there helping her, being part of this important move of hers. I hadn't even seen her new apartment. When will I get to see it? Will I ever be out of this place?

Because of the move, Mother had fallen behind in keeping my nails trimmed. When Gerda and Wim made their weekly stop, Gerda noticed that my nails were getting too long. "Oh, Sue," she said, "next time I come I'll bring my manicure set and do them for you." The offer was kind, but I had to stop her. It would upset Mother to have someone else take over the one thing she treasured doing for me. This had become her special gift of love. Bill would have to straighten this out.

Tell Gerda Mother does nails. Bill studied the words he wrote in his book, then looked at my nails, even more puzzled. *Tell Mother come do nails before Gerda comes back.* Now he understood. He smiled and shook his head benignly. Much ado, I could imagine him thinking. But he would take care of it.

The next day Mother came with her equipment. "I'm sorry I let them get so long, Sue. I hadn't realized how fast your nails grow."

The feelings inside were warm and sincere as she manipulated each finger and toe, clipping and filing. "Well, look at that, the calluses are getting thinner, just as I promised. They'll all be gone by the time you start . . ." Her voice cracked. I could hear the tears, though she never looked up. ". . . when you start walking again." She wrapped her tools in a tissue and put them in her purse, still struggling for composure. Yes, Mother, I will walk again. I know I will. And it will be wonderful not to have those troublesome calluses. Our tears commingled as she kissed me and left, unable to say good-bye.

I worried about Mother now. She'd had troubles before and always handled them beautifully, without complaint. She fought back, and everyone admired her ability to cope. But now she was shut off from real communication with me and felt closed off from Bill as well. Still she tried to keep the right foot forward when she was with me, just as she'd done with the whole world when Daddy was sick.

When Mother visited during the week, Bill was always there. I could communicate readily with him, and there was a lot to be spelled to him. I could see that she felt left out, but what could I do? She would pat my foot or leg all the while she was there, transmitting her feelings of helplessness over not being able to do anything to make me better.

Mother tried to hide anything bad from me, but she wasn't successful. If she had an upsetting day or was particularly unnerved by seeing me, I always knew it. It showed all too clearly in her eyes, even in her posture. Some days she left very quickly—to go outside and have a good cry. But always I knew.

Mother's feeling of exclusion troubled me. Bill had always gotten along very well with my mother, but he was so busy taking care of me and everything at home that there wasn't time or opportunity to offer her any support. He was barely getting through each day himself. Yet she needed him, and he needed her. Each was so afraid of upsetting the other that they did nothing to reach out and share their pain. So, except for our Saturday mornings and occasional Sundays when she was alone with me, I could see that Mother felt shut out, and I knew of no way to undo the situation. Oh, please, God, I must get out of here and back to my family again.

"February 10: 10 weeks. Mouth saliva always problem. Coughing."
—from Bill's diary

Visitors were such a blessing. My friend Jo from church still came regularly—often with another member of the congregation. Tonight she arrived with Ruth. Immediately my cubicle radiated with Ruth, a warm, expansive person who spreads love wherever she goes.

"Hello, honey," she said with her usual sincerity. To Ruth, everyone is always a sweetie, or dear, or honey. Normally, she also freely administers hugs or a kiss. But after studying my tubes and wires for an instant, she settled for a warm hand embrace. Jo stood quietly at the foot of the bed, enjoying Ruth.

"My, we have missed you at church, dear." Immediately, as

she talked, Ruth reached for a washcloth, wet it, and began wiping off my face. I remembered that she was trained as a nurse. "But we're all keeping posted on your progress every Sunday. Sam gives us a weekly report." The washcloth felt so good. Her touch was perfect, firm enough to clean off the perspiration and drooled saliva, yet nonabrasive. Ruth, that feels so good!

As Ruth moved from one side of the bed to the other, Jo stepped up to the bed. Her smile and handclasp were so warm that she needed no words. We both just listened to Ruth's pleasant monologue.

Ruth finished washing my face and pulled at a loose corner of the sheet, drawing out all the wrinkles. Hmm, could I possibly get her to do a little in-service training for the staff? "I try to catch Bill after service to ask about you, but he rushes out as fast as he can."

Comes here. Jo interpreted the spelling, as Ruth plumped the pillows at my back. "Of course. We all understand. Who wouldn't come rushing to you?" Her laughter was a delight. Then she sobered. "But we do worry about him, Sue. He never smiles, and he's looking a little thin."

Is thinner. Too busy. And certainly there isn't much for Bill Baier to smile about these days. All the while Jo translated and smiled warmly, her expression full of understanding and caring. Ruth replaced and fluffed the pillow under my head.

"There. Is that better?"

Yes. Thanks. Thank you so very much for noticing.

"Does Bill have anyone he can talk to, Sue?"

Me. Talks to me.

"Oh, I know, honey. Of course he talks to you. But I mean someone to really talk to."

I guess no one else could understand that from the very beginning of my illness, Bill shared everything with me, good and bad. If the car needed new tires, he'd say, "Sue, would you believe . . . ?" He'd tell me when the refrigerator broke down, or he was concerned about the girls—even about the hospital bills. Throughout our marriage, we have always shared everything, so now he just continued. This kept me from worrying just about myself and shifted some of my concern to the stresses Bill was facing.

As Ruth tugged on the sheet to get out one last wrinkle, Jo said softly, "Tell Bill we're here if he needs someone to talk to."

Yes. Yes, I would tell him. And I knew he would appreciate the offer. But Bill and I were both brought up believing that you keep your troubles to yourself, within the confines of the family. You don't tell the world. We were taught to be private. Everybody has problems, so you don't bother other people with yours. You handle them yourselves. Bill Baier would share his heartache where he always had—with me.

"Bye-bye, dearie," Ruth said, and this time she did find room for a hug, as Jo looked on, still smiling. "I'll be back soon, I promise." I hope so, Ruth. I hope you both come back soon. The contrasting radiance of the two, like a multicolored rainbow, lingered long after they left.

How fortunate we were to have an extended family like the people at St. Philip. Religion was important in my home as I was growing up, but since joining the congregation at St. Philip, our involvement had become more of a way of life than simply praying and Sunday churchgoing.

I was raised Methodist, but I married a man who already was a deacon in the Presbyterian church—at a young age. Bill grew up with a neighborhood church in New Jersey, and both of his parents were involved there. So when Bill came to Houston, it was natural for him to become involved in a congregation here. When I met him, I was impressed that as a single man he was an officer in his church. Our religions were similar, and while we dated, we visited each other's churches. But I was not settled into a community in Houston. Bill was. When we decided to get married, I felt it was important that we share this aspect of our lives. Differing religions could be a problem in a marriage, and there was no need for us to have that, so I chose to join the Presbyterian church. I think it bothered my parents a little, but they felt it was my decision to make. It is a decision I have never regretted.

Once we joined St. Philip, I eventually became involved in The Women of the Church, a group that sponsors a wide range of projects for various needy causes. Sometimes we have food drives, or we get together to roll bandages or make gowns for newborns. At Christmas we ask church families to prepare "seamen's boxes" for mariners who are staying at the Houston Seamen's Center between sailings—away from their families over the holidays. The contents are practical—a pair of socks, stationery, a pen, soap, a comb, toothpaste—anything that will let the men and women know someone in Houston cares about them at Christmastime. Through The Women of the Church, I have made many friends, such as Jo and Ruth.

How I missed going to church with Bill now. I was always proud and happy to stand beside him during services. And I missed our couples' Sunday-school class. We have been with the same group since we came to St. Philip. The members are all so stimulating, and our studies of current issues, as they related to Scriptural teachings, have broadened my perspectives immeasurably.

The visit from Jo and Ruth again made me realize how much I missed all those wonderful people who have become such a large and important part of our lives.

Any part of me that moved even a little was encouraging. One day I found I could move one big toe up and down ever so slightly. I could hardly wait to tell Bill that something else moved, at last. He studied the toe from several angles, obviously intrigued. Was a new idea taking shape? Nearly every day I complained to him that people still were ignoring me and my sleighbells, so his mind was back to work on the problem. Before long, he walked in smiling.

"I think I have an alarm system for you." He was holding an old-fashioned brass alarm clock, the kind with the two big bells on top. Everyone standing nearby stopped to watch. They knew Bill was a no-nonsense person, and they really seemed to respect him.

"For the system to work," Bill explained, "the clock must never be wound." As he spoke, he glanced at his audience, checking to see whether they were listening. "The alarm must be set to the same time as the clock." Then he wound the alarm only, showing everyone that there was tape over the winding button of the clock. Next he removed a length of string from his pocket, tied it to the alarm switch, and then pinned it to the sheet to keep it taut. I could visualize what was coming next and laughed to myself as he tied the other end of the string to my toe.

"There. Now, Sue, move your toe."

Still smiling to myself, I waited for an imaginary drum roll. Then I consciously moved my toe forward. It triggered the clock's alarm lever, and you could hear it all over ICU! Those who weren't already watching came over to see what was happening. There was laughter and clapping. What a relief to have a "call button" that would command attention. Bill was obviously pleased that his idea worked and that the staff was enthusiastic about it. But he soon sobered, knowing he had to get his message across to everyone. Running his hand along the string, he reiterated the process.

"Once the alarm runs down, someone has to turn off the switch, rewind the alarm, and reset it." Everyone nodded agreement. But already I could name the staff members who would remember and those who would forget—on this shift alone. Plus there were two other shifts and all the relief people.

For a few days, "Sue's alarm" intrigued everyone and became quite a topic of conversation. As new people came on duty and saw the shiny brass clock, some even asked about it. They studied the system and gladly learned how to do it. Others were shown how to use it but never did. Still others just shrugged and ignored it.

But at least I had a way of getting attention.

If the clock was wound, Bill explained, it would kill the system—thus the piece of tape over the clock-winding stem. Some still couldn't understand, however. I watched helplessly as Louise tore off the tape. "There," she said proudly, winding the clock, "now it will work. Can't set off an alarm without the clock being wound, too." For once, she even managed to trigger it properly—to make it go off every time the clock arrived at the alarm time! Fortunately, Kay noticed the ticking clock, and she turned off the alarm switch. But I was without my signal until the clock ran down twenty-four hours later.

Like the bells, this alarm, also, was something I did not use unless someone I could trust was available. The night after Bill brought in the alarm, Aurilla was my nurse. Bill very carefully described the system to her. Later, when I desperately needed turning, I triggered it to call her. She came running, her arms waving. It upset her, just as all the monitor alarms did, and she started fooling with the respirator, thinking it was causing the noise. Then she walked off, with the alarm still jangling until it ran down. She hadn't asked me what I wanted—she just fouled up the dials of the respirator. Now I remained uncomfortable, needing turning and a respirator adjustment, until I could signal a therapist to reset it.

For over two months, I wore gowns with the same little blue print. I was so tired of that "feed-sack" print, and wearing the same thing day after day. Every once in a while I noticed a gown with a different pattern in the clean laundry stack that was rolled by my cubicle. One day Harriet pulled out one—a yellow and green model—for me.

How nice . . . a change!

I felt I'd been in a prison uniform all this time, depressed by the awful sameness—as well as by my greasy hair and perspiring face. Finally, I had a different gown! Silly, perhaps, that something so minor could mean so much, but for me, the whole world had drawn into smaller, narrower focus.

Even Bill noticed the "new" gown when he came. His eyes lit up. "You're wearing something different!" That was a look I hadn't seen for a long time. It almost made me feel feminine again. I love pretty clothes and make most of my own. It has always been fun to model something new for Bill. He's a very frank reviewer. His enthusiastic response now was indicative of just how long I'd worn that same tired pattern.

The different gowns—left over from separate purchase orders—came in a variety of patterns. Several of the morning nurses began going through the laundry each day when it came in, and if there was one different gown, they slipped it stealthily into my cubicle. At least twice a week, I got a different gown. Hallelujah!

Katherine's ski trip was scheduled for the midterm break. I began to wonder if she had everything she needed, but it was impossible for me to be of much help in getting her ready. My questions, as usual, went to Bill and then long distance to Katherine. Surely Elizabeth would have given her suggestions, too.

I had to keep telling myself that Katherine was a big girl, living away from home. She could take care of herself. Perhaps my apprehensions derived partly from being a nonskier. Still, I was pleased that the girls were having these opportunities. All that snow, of course, was exciting for my Houstonian daughters. Katherine did not remember her first blizzard in New Jersey, and measurable snow on the ground was rare in Houston, but they both remembered snow in Europe.

The year we lived in Holland, we were sure they'd see a snowfall, but Holland had an extraordinarily warm winter. Friends told us it snowed three times that year in Houston, but there was none in The Hague. So we decided to search out some snow. At Thanksgiving, we traveled to West Berlin. It was frightfully cold and there was ice on the ground, but no snow. One afternoon we lost ourselves for hours in a fabulous museum, a small version of the Smithsonian. All of a sudden, Bill and I looked out of a window and saw that it was snowing! We grabbed the girls and rushed to the windows.

The guards looked at us sternly. This was not a tourist time of year, and we probably were the only Americans there. Bill explained to them in his best German that this was the first time our children had seen snow. The guards smiled, probably bewildered about people who didn't see snow in the winter.

The sweetness of that reverie was halted abruptly. Suddenly, instead of snow, I saw again in my memory the people of East

Berlin, and I recalled watching them on our bus tour into the Eastern Sector. They seemed to be a country of prisoners. Tears came to my eyes then, and again now, as I look around me. Now I am a prisoner, just like them.

From my bed I watched the other "prisoners" across the way. I knew pretty well what was wrong with each of them. Some I could diagnose by the procedures being done. Others I learned about from the nurses talking across my bed. On my side of the room I could only hear the patients, not see them.

In the next cubicle was an older woman—she sounded very grandmotherly. I didn't know what was wrong with her, but she obviously was somewhat confused. During the day shift, most of the nurses were very kind to her, gentle and loving. If she tried to get out of bed, which happened occasionally, they went in to her and said, "Now, Mrs. Born, let us help you turn. You don't want to get out of bed right now." And they would ease her right back into bed.

But when Bruce came on duty, he had his studying to do. I heard him tell her he was putting her in restraints because she wasn't supposed to get out of bed. This really upset me because he was the only one who did it. It seemed to me such a cruel way to treat someone so powerless.

I thought back to my own maternal grandmother, for whom I was named, feeling grateful that she had kept her full faculties as long as she lived. Mama Sue, as everyone called her, was a charming, vibrant woman right up until she died at eighty-nine.

She and I were very close. When she heard I was getting married, she told Mother, "I don't know what I'm going to do if I don't like this young man." She didn't think there was anyone good enough for her granddaughter. Then Bill met her. He smiled and gave her a big hug. "I haven't had a grandmother in a long time," he said, "and now I have one again." Of course, she just melted.

Mama Sue lived in Fort Worth for many years, and when she was about eighty-seven, we planned to stop off and visit her one weekend, en route to the Six Flags over Texas amusement park.

When we stopped to see her at the retirement home, she was determined to go with us. So we decided it would be fun to take her on some of the easy rides in the morning and then take her home for lunch and a nap while we went back to the park. No way. She wanted to go on everything.

I hoped that when Mrs. Born in the next bed got better, her confusion would clear up. I wanted her to be able to go to Six Flags with her great-grandchildren and enjoy life as Mama Sue had.

Eventually, Mrs. Born and most of the others left ICU. I was happy for them, but I always felt envious and forsaken as I watched each one being rolled out in a wheelchair.

The first time I was put into a wheelchair, it was not to leave ICU. Whoever decided such things had ordered that I be placed in an upright position to start building my strength. I was excited and frightened. Charles first showed me the chair, which was soon dubbed "Sue's Cadillac." It was an old-fashioned wooden wheelchair that looked rather like a high-backed arm-chair. It had a footrest and many elevation levels. Charles explained that it could be straightened out nearly horizontal so I could rest in it, and then it could be pulled back up again to various angles of straightness, almost like a lawn chair. It was a monstrously awkward relic, but it was to be mine for many months.

With much reassuring, Charles sat me up in bed and then slowly lifted me to the chair. Ginnie and Carol carefully checked and secured all my tubes and connections. What a chore! I was settled on one pillow, with another behind my head, and then strapped into place with a pair of seatbelts. My limp body felt scarily insecure. I was sure I would fall over. Still, I was sitting up! All the ICU staff applauded the big move.

The first day I lasted thirty minutes, and Ginnie stayed with me the whole time. To everyone's surprise, I didn't get dizzy— apparently extraordinary after all those weeks of lying prone. But the bed felt good when Charles settled me back into it. Tomorrow, Charles said, they'd let me sit up a little longer.

Wonderful! Another step forward. Then I heard them saying that after this I could be left sitting up alone. That I did *not* like to hear.

The next day, however, I was introduced to Dick, a young man just starting his training in physical therapy. One of Dick's first assignments was to sit with me while I was in the chair. Dick was a part-time college student, bright and pleasant, and he was willing to spell with me, especially about our mutual interest: the Houston Rockets basketball team. I was relieved to have him nearby.

While sitting up, I finally could see my legs and arms. It was a ghastly sight. I was literally skin and bones—Charles estimated that I probably weighed eighty-five pounds. Bones protruded everywhere. They were a problem when I was lying down, but they were far worse when I was sitting, for my weight was concentrated on a small area. After just a few minutes in the chair, my hip bones jabbed through the thin layer of skin. *Hurts*, I spelled with Dick, and, bless his heart, he tried to move me to make it easier. He was kind and conscientious.

My fear lessened, but the pain increased. Each day, my time in the wheelchair was longer and more uncomfortable—more painful. Ginnie was the only one who seemed to understand how much I hurt. Whenever it was time for the chair, she came in with an extra pillow or piece of foam. One day she had me up so high that I almost wobbled out of the chair. We all laughed.

The staff became convinced that I was afraid of the chair, fearful I couldn't breathe sitting up. Though breathing was more difficult, it was the pain that caused the anxiety. I liked being up. It was good to see the world from another position. This was the first time I was able to see the wall behind my bed! I also knew it was good for me to be up, building strength. But there was no way to tell anyone how much it hurt. The soreness never left me.

Moving me was an ordeal, requiring three or four people to lift me and handle all the sensors, the respirator, and the tubes. I never felt uneasy during the move, though; these therapists were the people I trusted. Yet it always hurt.

My time in the chair eventually increased to forty-five minutes, and by mid-February, I was at 2½ hours. I was pleased with my progress, but the pain had become excruciating. And I was being left alone—with nobody to talk to, not even the TV or radio to distract me. The novelty had worn off; the cheering was over. I had faded into the environment so thoroughly that no one even saw me.

I'd met Jane through The Women of the Church, but I was surprised she had time to visit me. I knew how busy she must be since starting back to school for a degree in nursing. Even more surprising, someone had taught her how to spell with me.

"What's exciting, Sue, is that right now we're studying Guillain-Barré." She had many questions. Would I mind answering them?

No.

"Was there anything besides your eyes that you kept control over?"

No.

"Did you ever lose the movement of your eyelids?"

Once. Benadryl overdose.

"Are you still getting your monthly cycles?"

No.

"That's probably because of your drastic weight loss. Do you feel tired most of the time?"

Exhausted all the time. Never enough rest.

"That's the most common symptom, besides the paralysis, among all Guillain-Barré patients, they tell us."

Question after question poured out. Often she had explanations to give me. How wonderful that this disease is now part of the course of study for nurses' training. Most of my nurses did not know anything about these symptoms and what they meant.

As we talked, Jane's eyes scanned the cubicle and the entire unit. She was doing her rotation in intensive care, and she observed everything around us, questioning anything different from what she was seeing in her ICU training. This was fun.

Jane was so happy in her nursing studies. I wondered what happens to make some nurses lose interest and dedication. I saw more joy in the faces of the people who picked cotton around

Richmond and Rosenberg when I was a girl than I saw here. And picking cotton was terrible work, as I learned during my very brief career in it.

During the summer after my freshman year in high school, I found my purse empty and wanted to buy a birthday present for the boy I was dating. A neighboring farmer leased the land around our house, and every summer he brought in workers to pick his cotton. I found out how much they were paid for a sack of cotton and I watched them scoot up and down those rows, pulling that cotton and filling their sacks. That looked like a good way to earn some money. Well, Mother and Daddy were horrified. "You can get money another way," they said. But the more they balked, the more insistent I became.

Mother tried reason. "It would be very awkward for the farmer because you are our daughter."

Finally they decided that the best way to teach me was to let me do it. However, because I sunburn easily and because my knees were unaccustomed to crawling, they sent me off to the fields with a big sun hat, knee pads, jeans that reached below my shoes, and a long-sleeved shirt. I was a sight! Of course, they sent a lunch along with me, so I could eat with the other pickers rather than come home at noon.

My family kept watch from the windows of our cool house. I knew they were watching, so I put up a strong front. I had to show them! But it was miserably hot, I was always dripping wet, and the work was hard. I stuck it out the better part of a day and filled my sack, earning $13. Then I was finished. But in that one day I learned a lot about hard work. It amazed me how people could be pleasant and cheerful under such unpleasant working conditions.

Within the next few years, the work was taken over by picking machines. That seemed like a wonderful invention— except perhaps for the people who needed to do that field work for something more basic than a birthday present for a friend.

Hooray! Subclavian came out!

I was glad to be able to tell Bill this good news. The subclavian had been my IV for two months, a long time. I felt enormous relief, not only to be rid of the tube, but to be rid of the pesky sensor attachment that so often set off the monitor alarm. And the next day, another benchmark: I was quite sure I could swallow just a little bit.

On Valentine's Day, Bill came in carrying a "card" from Elizabeth. She'd used the largest-size posterboard available, bright red, and cut out colored pictures of flowers from magazines, pasting them in the shape of a heart onto the board. It read simply, "Happy Valentine's Day." I hadn't seen any of her handiwork for so long. This was fun. It stayed on the wall until I left ICU and always drew attention. The mail was unusually heavy this day, and of course there was another Snoopy card, compliments of George and Hure. But there was also a sadness, a special loneliness I couldn't seem to shake.

Valentine's Day is always sentimental for me because it is the day Bill gave me my engagement ring. We had started dating in September, and on Christmas Day he asked my father for my hand. But we decided to keep our news a secret until I got a ring.

On Valentine's Day, we had planned to attend the symphony, but it started snowing and the streets iced over quickly. Bill called me while we were still at work and said he refused to go out on downtown streets that night because Houstonians don't know how to drive in such weather. He didn't mention that he was working on a plan for us to have a nice, quiet evening so he could give me an engagement ring.

While he was busily plotting his strategy, I decided that we couldn't just stay home on Valentine's night, so I called Chickie. "We've canceled our plans. How would you like to get up a bridge game?"

Bill was not too thrilled when I informed him cheerfully of "our" plans. Not only was he not an avid bridge player, but he had other things on his mind for the evening. Later that night, after the bridge game, he did give me my ring. I was so excited I couldn't speak. We were really engaged now! And I had a wedding to plan. I was going to marry this handsome, gentle, dear man and become Mrs. William E. Baier, Jr. What a lovely sound that name had!

Now that I was sitting up in the wheelchair, I could look at my bare third finger. I missed wearing my rings and I felt angry with Bruce all over again. I knew the rules, but knowing them didn't help. Whenever a female took care of me, I looked for rings, and I silently and sadly admired all engagement and wedding rings.

I was terribly upset when Carol told me she'd lost her wedding ring down her bathroom sink. Each day I asked about it. She called a plumber to take the trap apart in hopes of finding it, but it was lost. At least my rings were waiting for me in the safe-deposit box.

"February 15: Talk to the lawyer about the will—if Sue incapacitated, provision for everything to be taken care of."
                                                          —*from Bill's diary*

Bill had his hands behind his back as he walked toward my bed. As always, I was watching the clock this morning. Last night had been bad. Lately, every night was bad—little time for sleep, but always horrifying dreams.

I couldn't believe my eyes. Bill was actually smiling, that smile I fell in love with. At the foot of the bed he paused, eyeing me mischievously. Then suddenly he pulled his hand in front of him, and I saw it—one tall, slender narcissus. My eyes filled with tears—loving, melancholy tears. Bill understood and kissed me.

"Happy spring, Sue." The words dissolved me completely. It was our annual ritual—usually I was the one to discover and coddle the first spike of new growth. This year it was Bill's turn.

We'd had the bulbs sent from Holland to be a special, living reminder of our spring in The Hague. They were our signal of spring, Houston's beautiful February spring. Oh, Bill, dare we hope that our lives are also coming into spring, a time of rebirth? How I want to go home with you, Bill. The silent words passed through our eyes. Bill's second good-morning kiss told me he understood.

Even Penny, a Zeta sorority sister, must have sensed it was a special day. She sent me a big bunch of colored balloons—something not yet popular in Houston—with a note saying she'd thought about me a lot and felt helpless because she couldn't do anything for me. What a misstatement. Those balloons delighted me. Penny was someone I'd served on committees with, but I didn't know her well. Yet she gave me this buoyant gift.

Soon after Harriet tied the balloons to the side of the bed, another nurse walked in and said, "We can't have these in intensive care." And off she went with my balloons! I was devastated.

Harriet noticed that they were gone as soon as she got back from lunch. "Where are your balloons?" I glared at the nurses' station. Off she went in a fury and returned with them in a few minutes. "You may not be able to have plants, but these balloons are not going to hurt a single, solitary thing," she announced with determination. She tied them at the foot of the bed, where I had a good view of them. And there they remained. Every time I opened my eyes, they made me feel like smiling. I couldn't tell anyone what they did for me. They gave me a double boost—because Penny thought of sending them and because Harriet went to bat for me. Everyone came in and teased me about them. When the helium failed, they just draped the limp balloons over the side of the bed and finally hung them on the curtain.

"February 18: People saying I look like I'm aging."
—from Bill's diary

Elizabeth brought me her invitation to the spring Cotillion— always a lovely, special dance for girls from the various high schools in West Houston. She knew I would be interested because I was a member of the Cotillion board and had planned and helped with several functions. Immediately my mind raced into gear. She'll need a new formal.

Before I could jump too far ahead, I saw the look on Elizabeth's face. "Did you read it?" she asked indignantly.

I hadn't had time, but she was still holding the invitation in front of my face.

"Can you believe it? The Cotillion is having a 'kicker' dance," she said. I hadn't noticed. I'd been concentrating on the date. I read it. It was to be a country/western "kicker" dance. Her expression was a mixture of disdain and disappointment. I couldn't blame her. Elizabeth loved dances, but country/western was not her favorite. They were all right for club parties, but certainly not for the Cotillion. To Katherine, "kickers" were the best way to go, but Elizabeth liked formals. How different these girls are!

"Oh, Mother, this just isn't right." I knew what she was leaving unsaid—if I'd been at the board meeting, I might have been able to change their minds. Well, I'm not there this year, Elizabeth. You'll just have to pull on your jeans and go have fun. At least I didn't have to worry about a long dress for her. Still, I'd love to have that formal to worry about.

Dressing my girls has always been pure joy for me. When they were little, I took great pride in their appearances. I polished their little saddle oxfords every night. It seems I spent my life back then whitening scuffed toes. When the three of us were out, people smiled at them and even stopped to compliment me on my daughters. One woman approached me in a department store to say, "Excuse me, but may I tell you how loved your children look? I can tell by looking at them how you care for them."

They sometimes enjoyed having matching clothes when they were in lower elementary school. One spring, I bought them twin outfits with red blazers, blue-and-white-striped knit tops, and blue pleated skirts. I even found red-and-blue dress shoes to match. Many people commented on those outfits, and I was proud of them. I still love shopping with them for their clothes. It would be fun to look for a Cotillion gown now for Elizabeth, but we were both to be disappointed.

I was getting so tired I could scarcely face each new day. Therapy was becoming more extensive, and then there were breathing treatments, feedings, and all the hours sitting in the chair. The pain in my abraded hips never stopped, and it sapped my strength.

I was often left alone in that chair for three hours at a time, staring in whatever direction I'd been pointed. The frustration, boredom, and pain were totally exhausting. Life here in ICU was like a roller coaster—highs and lows. But the lows were getting deeper. Was there a bottom?

I was concerned about my ability to handle everything much longer. There had to be something to give me the energy to make it through the day.

Need vitamins.

So Bill talked to Dr. Lohmann, and he ordered vitamins. Why doesn't anyone else think of these things? Must I be my own doctor, too?

"February 22: Looks bad. Feeling of dread."

—from Bill's diary

I didn't like taking tranquilizers, but whenever I got upset, they administered them. I had to get some of the frustrations removed if I was to avoid getting them. And Aurilla was my biggest single frustration. She was *always* there.

I had to get through to Bill somehow. But whenever I complained, he just sighed in resignation and dutifully wrote the complaints in his book.

Since Aurilla upsets me, why can't we get her off? Can't communicate, suction. When I sweat, why can't they wipe me off? Will need more Valium.

The words were becoming too familiar now for Bill. Just as the staff no longer saw me, Bill no longer was hearing me. Even as he wrote the words in his book, they became invisible to him, too. I saw it in his face and I felt betrayed. He was the only one I had to help me.

"February 26: Lohmann says: Blood gases not good. Infection. Antibiotics begun. Birmingham says: In one or two months, we will sit over a good drink and smile."

—from Bill's diary

13

Some mornings were worse than others. Today I was very low. Will this really ever end?

"Good morning. I'm Paulette, your nurse today." Oh, no, another new person! I can't deal with anyone new today. "I'll be back in a little while with your bath."

Another new nurse.

By now Bill dreaded new staff as much as I did, and he especially disliked getting bad news first thing in the morning. Immediately he called her over to explain how to spell with me. She seemed to understand. That was a hopeful sign.

After Bill left for work, Paulette returned, as promised. She began my bath, and I knew immediately she sensed everything I was feeling. Her warm, brown face smiled kindly, empathetically. She was efficient and thorough. My goodness, she's wonderful, I kept repeating to myself. Where did she come from? She had the maturity to understand what I needed and the skills to make me comfortable.

By the time Bill came at noon, I could hardly wait to tell him. *Feeling better. Nurse Paulette really good.*

He shared my elation. If only I could have her every day, intensive care just might be tolerable.

But good news seldom could be savored for very long. A new blow: Kay was leaving to accept a position in respiratory therapy at another hospital. She had received such a good offer, she said. But all I could think was, How could she leave? She's been my overnight life-saver. I was devastated.

That evening Bruce had me, and, noticing my teeth were discolored, he decided to do something about them. Apparently they had become discolored because of lack of good, regular cleaning and the constant stagnant saliva accumulating around the teeth and gums.

167

"I'm going to clean your mouth with peroxide," he said. Surely he can't mean that. I watched in disbelief as he plunged a large swab into the bottle—pure peroxide—and suddenly he began gouging, forcibly jabbing the peroxide-soaked swab into my mouth and into my gums and teeth. I screamed silently in agony and rage. And I became frightened. Could he read the expression in my eyes? I fought not to show any sign of disapproval, because the more upset I would become with him, the rougher he would get.

"I'm just doing this for your own good. Your teeth need cleaning," he said flatly, forcing my lips to stay apart. The peroxide frothed from my mouth; its vile taste gagged me and burned every crevice. Still he slammed and jabbed the swab into my teeth and gums. My eyes filled with involuntary tears. Moments seemed hours as I fought off hysteria. Finally he stopped, but the pain and burning did not.

I watched the hands of the clock, waiting for Bill. He promised he'd come back tonight. Where was he?

Before I could begin spelling, Bill recognized the look in my eyes. Tears rolled down my cheeks as I responded to each letter. Bill's face turned red, then ashen. He wheeled around in a sweep of anger and called Mary Jean. This was the first time he had ever called her to the bed.

"Look what Bruce did. He cleaned Sue's teeth with pure peroxide. He was rough, and he hurt her. Look at how upset she is."

Even Mary Jean was taken aback. Another first: In front of us, she said to Bruce, "Please don't do that to her again." Then she turned to me and said, sweetly, "But, Sue, he did mean well."

Don't tell me that. I don't want to hear any more about people meaning well. I am a patient. I am a human being. It costs nothing to be kind and understanding—to dilute peroxide, if it must be used, and to be gentle and reassuring. I am tired of trying to understand people who "mean well." It was hard to hold back the tears. Gently Bill dried my eyes, wiped out my mouth with tissue, freshened it with a half-dozen sixty-cent lemon swabs!

After Bill left, I drew some comfort in realizing that this was the first time anything bad had been halted at the start. For the first time I saw Bill Baier take a stand with me against them. Three cheers for Bill!

Later, Bruce came to turn me. There was no recognizable expression in his eyes or in his voice. "Your teeth needed it, you know. Now it's done."

With growing concern now, I watched my fellow patients from my silent perch. I watched their nursing care—some good, some bad, and some that was heroic. . . .

Paulette was always terrific, both with me and with others. She seemed easygoing, yet a real perfectionist. She even looked like someone who did everything well.

One day, as Paulette was going off duty at three o'clock, the nurses were having difficulty stabilizing a patient on the other side of the unit. They had called several codes for him already. The head nurse asked Paulette to stay for another shift, just to look after this patient. For eight hours she fought for his life, and I fought silently with her, wanting her to win. I watched her use electric shock paddles to revive him. Then she worked on his chest with her hands—anything to bring him back and keep him going. She had worked hard for eight hours with me and her other patients, plus the codes, and now she was repeatedly reviving him. I knew how exhausted she must be, but she never gave up.

Finally, at eleven, Paulette had to leave. An intense sixteen hours had left her visibly exhausted. I watched the next nurse come on duty, but she didn't seem to tend him with as much determination. I supposed the man was ready to die, anyway, and he did—shortly after the new nurse came on. It probably wasn't her fault, but it upset me that he died after all of Paulette's efforts. When they pulled the equipment away from his bed to make room for the stretcher bearers, I cried. If Paulette were still here, would he have lived?

"March 3: Shortage of nurses and therapists."
                                                  —*from Bill's diary*

Another new respiratory therapist—Don. He was frighteningly rough. He was from an agency—by now I knew that only agency people wore name tags. The first time he had me, he was abrupt. He jerked my head into position and suctioned me, without doing it completely. Here we go again.

But Don did spell with me. And a miracle happened: I told him he was rough, and he changed!

He told me one evening later that he became a respiratory therapist because he was nearly killed in an automobile accident. He'd "been there"—ICU, respirator, everything. After he came out of it, he decided this was something he had to do. And from that first night, he never objected to my calling him on something or reminding him of a missed procedure. When Earl, the director of respiratory therapy, came to check me, which he did periodically, I made sure to tell him about Don. I wanted him to be called for relief work whenever possible.

Don talked about his children. When he saw I was interested, he told me about his divorce and the fact that his wife had taken their children to El Paso. He brought in their pictures for me to see. I knew when he had talked to his children and when he was disappointed because he hadn't been able to. But his disappointments never detracted from his work. Often he spoke of his loneliness and a feeling of isolation. These were emotions I knew, and he seemed to understand that.

Something strange was going on with my case, and I was trying to put the pieces together.

Funny. Birmingham, Gary, and Earl—each one—says he's in charge. Bill, too, was noticing this.

Finally, we began to see the picture. All three—an anesthesiologist and the heads of the physical therapy and respiratory therapy departments—were telling the staff what to do. Each one was now telling me—and Bill—"I'm in charge. You listen to me and not the other two." Yet none of these men was the internist on the case. Dr. Lohmann still came every day, read my chart, and issued orders. But now there were other orders, issued by Birmingham—the one I wondered about most. His role in my care was still very fuzzy in my mind.

Bill would corner each of them, including Gary and Earl, whenever he could, trying to determine some strategy, some course of action for my care. Each man always came across as caring and confident about the outcome of my case, although they all recognized conflicts in my care program. Gary said too many things were interfering with my physical therapy program, which was true. No one wanted to set a schedule with PT, so therapy had to be worked in whenever possible.

Respiratory therapists seemed to be doing their part, and that had to come first. I had to get off the machine to get well. Earl assured Bill that I was right on schedule with my breathing. He was on top of the situation.

But Dr. Birmingham was always an unknown factor. He had his own strategy worked out for me, he said. Bill should leave everything to him.

All of this was upsetting Bill, but he didn't know what to do. He kept asking each of them, "What's your plan? What do you foresee happening when she comes off the respirator? Or when she gets over this infection? What have you worked out?" Supposedly all of these people were meeting together to assess my case and plan strategy. In fact, they all met together with Bill only once, each reporting what he was going to do. Then, each of them later talked to Bill reassuringly, saying virtually the same thing: "Now, don't worry. I'm in charge. I'll take care of everything." Bill could not relate to such irregular management practices. Who was in charge?

As for Dr. Lohmann, Bill didn't know what to make of him and his relationship with the others. The doctor did not seem to play a part in what the other three were doing or saying. I knew he was convinced that I was getting the best of care, but I could not figure out where he fit into all of this. He was my doctor, but he wasn't a part of the "trinity."

Dr. Lohmann greeted me every day in exactly the same pattern. "Hello, Sue." Then he'd reach for my radio and turn it off. "Let's turn this down while I'm talking to you." I'd wait, wondering if this finally was the day he was going to talk to me. He'd glance at the chart and ask the nurse a question or two.

"Did she sleep last night?"

"Yes, doctor, she had a good night," the nurse answers.

No. In fact, I didn't sleep at all. No one ever got me comfortable. But Dr. Lohmann never looks at me to see *my* answer.

"Any problems with the feedings?" he asks the nurse.

"No, doctor. . . ."

Yes. Yes, doctor. I have always had a small stomach. They're shoving so much of the supplement down me that sometimes I feel sick. Bill says I should just let it go sometime—throw it up all over them. But I just can't do that, doctor. Please, doctor, look at me and let me tell you.

He looks! I blink frantically to signal him that there's something I need to say.

"See what she wants, nurse." Then he is gone—and again, just like every other day, he has left my radio off. The nurse leaves with him.

"I'll be back in a few minutes, Sue," she says. But she won't. She'll be back when it's convenient for her—or in another hour, when it's time for my next feeding.

Why can't he try to communicate with me? And why is all this in-fighting going on over me? Who *is* in charge? How do any of the nurses and therapists know what to do when all these "in-charge" people don't know who is in command?

Only one member of the staff ever acknowledged this mounting chaos—my advocate, Charles. He was the one constant factor each weekday, a totally loyal champion in a world that seemed to have forgotten I was human.

Charles was "popping" my toes. This little procedure at the end of the leg and foot movements had become a kind of game of ours. He would pull each toe one by one so the knuckle popped. All the while, he'd look at me and smile, and his eyes would react with a little extra sparkle when each toe snapped. At first, I worried about this, remembering the old wives' tale that popping joints made them grow larger. My feet are big enough—how big will they be if he does this two or three times every day? But I knew that was nonsense, so I relaxed and enjoyed the experience, often singing to myself, "This little piggy went to market. . . ." Such a small silliness was often the bright spot of a bleak morning or afternoon.

"I am going on vacation, Sue, starting next week." Charles was trying to smile as he said it, but there was concern in his face. As his words sank in, terror seemed to make all my useless muscles recoil. I felt sick to my stomach and fought for control. *Yes. Stay calm, Sue.*

"It'll be all right, Sue. Ginnie and JoAnn will be here to take care of you, and I'll be back in two weeks." Charles read my eyes better than anyone at the hospital, so I made myself not cry, at least until he left. Then everything poured. How could I survive if Charles left me for two weeks? I trusted Ginnie and JoAnn, but Charles was so much a part of my day—from that first visit in the morning, carrying his cup of coffee, until the late-afternoon workout. He was the one staff person I always could count on. Now he'd be gone for two weeks. But I would survive, I assured myself. I had to.

"March 6: 7:00, Elizabeth dance pickup. Sue wants two visits."
                                    —*from Bill's diary*

Bill occasionally had a luncheon meeting and could not come in for the noon visit. In these rare instances he arranged with one of my friends to cover for him. Today it was Bess. I knew she was coming, and I was waiting eagerly for her when she arrived. I felt all smiles when she walked in.

However, right behind her was Gary Stiller. Bess looked as surprised as I was to see him.

"Sue, we're going to try something." I didn't like the sound of that—especially when I wanted to visit with Bess.

"We're going to take you off the machine for five minutes." My eyes darted to Bess. She looked as unsure as I felt. "We've been doing tests and we know you can stand it. You've already done two minutes." Fear mounted. That was different! I hadn't even known what was happening then, and two minutes is not five minutes. Besides, then I had Kay and Harriet. "All you have to do is blink when you want me to put you back on." That was a relief. Maybe I could handle it. "I would very much like for you to go five minutes if you can, but you don't have to."

I looked at Bess again. Her eyes were riveted on Gary. You fox, I thought. Bess is here, and he's tied this all together. He's using her visit so I won't protest. But why was he the one doing this? He was no longer head of the respiratory therapy department. Earl was.

Bess was at my side, clinging to my hand. Her touch and her eyes told me it would be all right. She'd make sure I got back on the respirator when I needed it.

Gary removed the respirator connection from my trach and attached the oxygen tube. I looked at the clock. I was annoyed that he played this game of using Bess, but I was determined to last the five minutes if I could. I'll show you, Gary Stiller. And if I can do it, if only I can do it, I'll be closer to getting off that machine for good.

I watched the clock, counting off seconds; one minute, then two. I glanced at Gary, who was checking his watch. Three-and-a-half minutes. Why wasn't Earl or Peter trying this? Another power play of Gary's, I decided.

The second hand slowly crossed the fourth minute, and I was still breathing on my own. I looked at Bess. Her hand squeezed mine, support that came from years of caring.

The seconds counted down, seeming almost to stop at times, but I made it! A surge of excitement came over me as we all ended the countdown together. Bess was laughing joyfully. Even Gary's voice had an edge of excitement to it.

"I knew you could do it, Sue. Five minutes! I knew you were ready. We just had to try you out and see." Then I realized that despite the battle to see who was boss, Gary had done what needed to be done. He'd just decided on his own that the time had come, and he'd been right.

"Now you'll be able to try longer times, Sue," Gary said. "It won't be long now and you'll be off the machine, I promise you." I had the feeling he might be right about that, too.

After Gary reconnected me to the respirator, he left. It was then I noticed Luana at the foot of the bed. She wasn't my nurse that day, but she was there rooting for me. "Oh, Sue, I'm going to call Bill!" She was so excited.

Finally Bess and I had some time alone together to spell and talk. We were both still giddy with excitement, and her news of family and friends flowed freely.

Suddenly, my eye caught a glimpse of a figure at the foot of my bed. There stood Bill Baier, looking proud and happy. I wanted to shout: Did you hear what I did? Obviously he had heard, and he read the delight in my eyes. It was a triumphant moment.

During her next visit, Bess told me, "That day, after you breathed alone, I was looking at you while we talked. Suddenly, I saw a glow come over your face. Even though you couldn't move a muscle, your face radiated the moment you saw Bill." I had felt the glow, but I couldn't imagine that anyone could see it. Only Bill makes me feel that way.

Charles returned from vacation, and I was eager to hear all about his trip. But first I had to show him my newest accomplishment—pulling in my stomach muscles.

"What on earth are you doing?" I had never seen Charles look so cross. Even Ginnie, who was with him, looked surprised.

Birmingham gave exercise for stomach. One day when Dr. Birmingham noticed that I could move my stomach muscles a tiny bit, he told me about an exercise I could do to strengthen those muscles. So I was doing it often on my own whenever I was alone and needed something to do. I was ready for anything that might strengthen my abdomen. I was sure Charles would be pleased.

"You are going to undo everything I've been working on," he said, almost shouting. "We don't need those muscles strengthened now. If they get overdeveloped, it will be harder for us to build up the back muscles when we try to sit you up."

Weeks later, Charles was still fighting those muscles I had worked so hard to develop.

Bill continued his efforts to sort out the problem of too many bosses. Perhaps it was the manager in Bill that directed his focus toward what was clearly a management problem. His diary was filling with notes about it: Talked to Birmingham. Talked to

Earl. Talked to Gary. Talked to Lohmann. Each had a different approach.

My latest and most urgent pleading had to do with scheduling. Fatigue was becoming more serious every day as more and more therapy was being done with me. I needed a little rest period between my bath and physical therapy. But there was no time for rest. No one was coordinating schedules among the various departments. I was caught in the middle of what seemed to be a tug-of-war.

Anger, exhaustion, depression. I felt locked in the unending cycle. The tears began to flow every time I saw Bill. He struggled through my spelling out every frustration, and whenever I cried, he cried. His anguish made mine even more unbearable.

Then finally came another breakthrough.

Day after day, I continued to monitor myself, testing every muscle from toe to head. Then I suspected something new was occurring, but I couldn't be sure. One day, I was conscious that it was happening. I felt myself swallow, just a tiny amount of saliva. For some time James had predicted that this was imminent, as he saw my gag reflexes slowly returning. But was this certain? Could I trust that it was going to continue? That awful morning when I awoke, unable to swallow, came back vividly in my thoughts. But I forced my mind to concentrate on the positive. I can swallow again!

I began to think about the taste of food. Dwelling on food was a luxury I had not allowed myself for many weeks. Only when some unthinking nurse came near me, eating a sandwich or a cookie, would I covet food. Then I'd be tormented for hours, craving the taste of something.

Elizabeth came in several days after that first real swallow. In the midst of one of her animated stories, Dr. Muenkel entered. I was surprised when he picked up my chart and studied it.

"What has she been given to eat or drink since she began swallowing?" he asked.

"Nothing, as far as I know," replied the nurse.

"If she can swallow, why aren't you giving her anything orally?" The nurse appeared a little bewildered. "Get her some ice chips." The thought of ice chips was magnificent. Elizabeth watched the scene curiously as the nurse left to get the ice.

Wonderful. Elizabeth smiled at me and then interpreted for the doctor.

"My mother likes the idea of having some ice. I think this will be a first since she got here three months ago." She looked back to me.

Yes.

"Well then, Sue, I wish I could offer you something more spectacular for your first taste," he said.

Just fine.

The nurse brought a cup of crushed ice and held it out, uncertain what to do with it. Dr. Muenkel took the cup from her, set it on the table, selected one small ice chip, and positioned it on my tongue. It was cold, wet, and fresh. After a moment of pleasure, I started thinking about my throat. A swallow is not something one can see, like the movement of a toe—an accomplishment that I still found pleasant to watch. I concentrated, closing my eyes to avoid distraction. Then I felt muscles move ever so slightly, and the drop of melted ice slid down my throat. My eyes flew open in excitement.

Elizabeth smiled quietly at me, and Dr. Muenkel grinned broadly at both of us. He turned to the nurse, who also caught some of the enthusiasm. "Now, give her a few chips every couple of hours—and anything else she feels she can swallow." She nodded. "Take care, Sue. And enjoy anything you feel like ordering."

I was delighted at this new step and pleased that Elizabeth could share the moment. So often she saw only the bad times, with any good news coming secondhand from Bill.

"I can't wait to tell Daddy," she said. "He needs some good news."

Yes, he does.

"I haven't told you, Mother, because I was afraid to worry you. . . ."

Yes?

"So often at night, after we eat, Daddy goes up to his room—

your room—and shuts himself off. Sometimes, often, I can hear him crying. Sometimes I go to the door and want to go in, but I don't know what to say to him—except that I know you're going to get well. He knows that, too, doesn't he, Mother?"

Yes. He knows. Yes, Elizabeth, he does. And it is his faith that has kept me going. But there's no way to explain to you what he is going through.

"Well, at least I have some good news for him today." Reaching carefully around the tubes, she hugged me. "I love you." I love you, too, Elizabeth. "See you later."

It was a comfortable time for rest.

When Bill came in that night, he wore a huge smile and carried a container of ice cream! It looked heavenly. I struggled to make the first tiny drop go down, but it just coated my mouth. Ice cream was not going to work. Bill tried a second and third dab, but it just clogged my mouth. The look of disappointment on Bill's face mirrored my feelings. I'm so sorry, Bill. I want to eat it, especially for you, but I can't. I love you for thinking of it. Please understand.

"March 7: I took ice cream. She didn't want it."
—*from Bill's diary*

14

My times off the respirator, breathing with only supportive oxygen, were stretching out. Finally, on March 9, I was off the respirator from early morning until evening. It was a milestone. The next day, I made a decision. I was going off the machine for good!

James came in to reconnect the respirator that evening.

No. I'm off machine!

His expression was jubilant. "Are you sure, Sue?"

Yes! The answer was emphatic, but suddenly I was struck with a twinge of doubt. *Leave machine here.*

"Changing your mind already?" His grin was all the challenge I needed.

No! There would be no change of mind now. Still, I needed the security of having it by me—just in case something went wrong. I'd had too many disappointments already. I would rest easier with the security of that now-silent machine next to my bed.

Rest, however, did not come that first night. I was afraid to go to sleep. Could I really continue breathing on my own—especially if I was asleep and unable to make myself take the next breath? All night I monitored my body—and studied the clock and the ceiling light.

I hated that light. I closed my eyes and tried to think about darkness. Light still shone through my closed eyelids. What was darkness like? I couldn't remember; I couldn't feel darkness any more. The one darkness I could visualize now was a memory of a long-ago episode when we had no lamps in the house. And that I remembered because Bill would never let me forget!

Before Bill and I started dating, he bought a house from a couple getting a divorce. They wanted to sell the place furnished, and that suited bachelor Bill just fine. It seemed like a good investment. As long as the furniture was functional, he wasn't particularly concerned with how it looked. When we became engaged, I got a lot of teasing about marrying Bill for his house. Actually, I thought it would be fun to start out in an apartment like all the other young couples we knew. I wasn't sure I was ready for the responsibilities of a three-bedroom, two-bathroom house. But we had the house, and I knew I was lucky.

But there was not a thing in the house that looked like me. It was furnished in ultra-modern style, something that might have worked in an office, but not a home—not my home. Of course, Bill thought it was wonderful that we had everything we could possibly need.

Right after we returned from our honeymoon and Bill went back to work, I studied those rooms. Suddenly I had what I thought was a wonderful idea. I called Goodwill Industries and asked them to come immediately. I gave them all the accessories—every picture off the walls and every lamp in the house. If I got rid of those things, I reasoned, I would have made a start at making the place feel homey. At the time, I didn't think I was being frivolous. I couldn't wait to show Bill what I'd done.

He stared at the walls and bare tables in utter disbelief, as if someone had just knocked the wind out of him. "Sue, how are we supposed to buy new ones?"

I hadn't thought about that. What a quick education I got in the cost of home furnishings!

After two nights of a totally dark living room, Mother and I went shopping and found a pair of lamps on sale, so we finally had some light. But the rest—pictures, accessories, and remaining lamps—came very gradually. As soon as I could, I bought a slipcover for the couch and stitched it on very carefully so it would look upholstered. It took me days to sew it by hand. Finally, the house began to look like me.

I looked around ICU again. The yellow wall, the clock, the light panels, the white acoustical ceiling tiles with the little holes. I wondered whether Goodwill would take the whole room!

Shallow though it was, my breathing never stopped that night. I could make it without the respirator! I could sleep and still breathe. Now I was ready to get out of intensive care and into a real hospital room. This was the main reason I made myself give up the respirator.

The next evening, Bill and I were still sharing our pleasure at my new forward step when Dr. Birmingham came up to my bed.

"Well, you're off the machine," he said. "Now you need to start eating."

Before I could react to what he was saying, he reached up to my nose, grabbed hold of the NG tube, and yanked it out brutally. A silent scream of pain and fear ripped through me. My eyes flew to Bill, pleading for help, but he could not move. He stood there stunned, anger and disbelief swirling across his face.

"Now you'll have to eat," Birmingham said smugly, as he turned and left.

Bill clasped my hand, perhaps as much from his own need as from mine. Here I was, still barely able to swallow melted ice chips—and yesterday, my first drops of iced tea—and Dr. Birmingham seemed to think that his fiat alone could make me do something I was unable to do. He still seemed to know nothing about this disease.

Bill tried to comfort me, but I could see his anxiety. I'd been complaining about too much dietary supplement for my stomach to handle. Now there would be nothing—and here I was still at eighty-some pounds.

I was startled to hear Bill's words. "I just wish that some day I could do to him what he did to you." His eyes were glistening with angry tears. "Don't worry, Sue. We'll get this thing straightened out, I promise." I know, Bill. I know you will.

When Donna came on, she looked at me, incredulous. I was thankful it was she—someone who would understand. "Sue, your tube's gone! What am I going to do? I have all these meds to get down you." Dr. Birmingham hadn't thought about that. All my medications and vitamins had to be ground up and mixed with fruit juice to get them down the tube.

The next morning, drop by drop, Gwenn was able to get half a glass of juice and two tiny spoonfuls of cooked cereal down my throat. But I gagged when the mashed pills were added to the juice. By noon, another doctor was recruited to replace the NG tube. I tried to block out the faces leaning over me, the voices, and the torturous scraping of the tube up through my nose, back down my throat, and into my stomach. When Dr. Lohmann read the chart, his only reaction was to shake his head slowly and order my dietary intake doubled. Oh, doctor, please don't. I needed the feedings, but I was already getting more than my stomach could tolerate. He departed, leaving the radio turned off, as always.

One bright spot of the day: the respirator was removed from my cubicle.

Respiratory therapists constantly checked my blood gases to see whether I was getting sufficient oxygen. Now they added tests of vital capacity, the volume of air I was breathing. My volume was weak and my breathing shallow. "Sue, breathe deeper," became the new operative words. I'd always heard that lecturers and opera stars learned to breathe deeply from the diaphragm to sustain good, rich tone, but I had never learned the technique. I always spoke from high in my chest. Now I was relearning to breathe and having to remind myself with each breath to draw in more deeply.

Sitting in the old, wooden wheelchair was becoming more difficult—the pain of the rigid, unyielding seat seemed to be worsening. And now, for some reason, it was harder to breathe while sitting up. No one listened to or believed my complaints. And I was still anxious about being left alone where I could not trigger the alarm clock to call for help. In the midst of all this staff, I was alone and ignored. Perspiration would pour off me, stimulated by my anxiety over the pain, the heat of the unit, and my general weakness. Was it only my imagination, or was I getting weaker?

I complained to Bill. *Left sitting two hours. Hurt. No alarm. Dripping wet. No one wiped perspiration. Ignored.* Bill faithfully wrote the words and nodded with understanding. Did he understand?

"March 13: Talk about negative attitude."
                                    —from Bill's diary

I begged Bill to get me out of ICU.

"Patience, Sue. You have to have patience."

No more patience. I'd been patient for nearly four months. I was ready now. After all, I was off the respirator.

"Sue, they have to make sure you're breathing well enough to stay off the respirator."

Others get out day after off machine. I saw them all around me—off one day, out the next.

"But they weren't on as long as you." Always the voice of reason. "Also, you're still paralyzed and have your trach. The floor nurses are not trained to deal with you—nor do they have the time to take care of you *and* all the other patients on the floor."

Has to be way. Must get out.

"The only way to do it is with private-duty nurses. Once they give the go-ahead to move you, we're going to have to get this all lined up. It will all take time. . . ."

I could tell there was more. Finally, it came. "Sue, I don't know if the insurance company will approve private nurses. And if they don't, well, you know we just can't afford. . . ." His voice broke, and I saw the tears. But I could not deal with that "if."

Fatigue became my enemy. I was tired, terribly exhausted all the time. I never had a complete night's sleep, and even when I rested reasonably during the night, it was never quite enough. Physical therapy was increasing, as were respiratory treatments for my lungs, along with the long periods in the chair. All of this was more than I had the strength to bear. There was no relief.

"March 15: Pneumonia. Antibiotics must be increased."
                                    —from Bill's diary

I knew I had a problem. Suddenly, every time I was suctioned, I felt the need for "bagging"—extra pushes of air from the

Ambu-bag. Peter, particularly, seemed bothered by this, and his doubt bothered me. He was afraid I would become dependent on the bag. I felt the fullness in my lungs, but I didn't have sufficient lung power to cough it up. My breathing was still shallow.

Dr. Lohmann was ordering chest X rays—and so was Dr. Birmingham. The technicians would roll in the X-ray machine, pull away the pillows, and slide the hard, cold plate under my back. Click, click—that was it. And off they'd go, leaving me in a rumpled heap. Perhaps an hour later, another technician would return with the other doctor's orders. Again the cold X-ray plate and the click, click. Doesn't anybody look at my chart and see that I have just had an X ray? The technicians had their aprons to shield them, but what about me? What was going to protect me from all these X rays?

I sank into despair when the respirator was rolled back into my cubicle. I had pneumonia, and they said it was likely to cause breathing problems. I had to go back on the machine. My tears were uncontrollable. I had come so close to escaping from ICU, and I *was* getting better. Now I was hooked to the machine again. Next came the IV in my arm. "Just a little touch of staph," I was told. "Nothing to worry about."

Bill struggled to look brave and positive, but with each visit, the tears in his eyes obliterated words. I could scarcely bear to look at him and see his sadness.

I hit bottom. Would there ever be an end to this? Would I ever get out of this mechanical horror? Was the "room upstairs" just a myth? Now I succumbed to the fought-off words of Bill's warning. Perhaps the insurance company would not cover private nursing. Was my passionate desire to leave this place based on fantasy alone? Despair and depression were smothering me.

Tears poured out again when San Williams stood beside my bed. Perhaps realizing there were no words capable of restoring my hope, he reached immediately for my book of psalms. Quietly, he began . . .

The Lord is my shepherd; I shall not want. He maketh me to lie down in green pastures: he leadeth me beside the still waters. He restoreth my soul: he leadeth me in the paths of righteousness for his name's sake. Yea, though I walk through the valley of the shadow of death, I will fear no evil: for thou art with me; thy rod and thy staff they comfort me. Thou preparest a table before me in the presence of mine enemies: thou anointest my head with oil; my cup runneth over. Surely goodness and mercy shall follow me all the days of my life: and I will dwell in the house of the Lord for ever.

The tears were drying on my cheeks now. San smiled softly and held my hand. The words echoed back through my mind over and over—"He maketh me to lie down in green pastures. . . ."

I felt a new serenity; fear and despair were bathed away with my tears. Now I was experiencing an inpouring of confidence that all of this would pass. San left as quietly as he arrived. "He leadeth me beside the still waters."

Katherine had more disappointing news at school, and that—like all other bad news—gave me something diverting to be concerned about. Her close friend, Kelly, was planning to leave school and move with her family to the Carolinas. Katherine was very disappointed. She and Kelly had a special friendship and planned to room together next year. By this time of the year, others had already settled on their roommates for next year. I wanted to talk with Katherine, to reassure her, and to give her some ideas about next year's living arrangements. But here I was again, helpless when my daughter needed me.

Then Linda came in to report on the ski trip she hosted for the girls in Colorado. "Katherine just took off on those skis," Linda said. "It was as if she'd been born on skis." Katherine never cared about her phys ed classes—an inclination she obviously inherited from me—so I'd been especially nervous about her going on the slopes the first time.

"Of the beginners," Linda said, "she did better than anyone. She was wonderful." She held up pictures of the girls for me to see. How happy Katherine looked with all of her friends!

This was just the medicine I needed, and surely Linda knew it. The photographs were permanently imprinted in my mind. Now, if Katherine can just handle this loss of Kelly. . . . All right, Sue Baier, I lectured myself, if Katherine can handle skiing, she can handle anything else, including finding a new roommate.

"March 19: Birmingham orders IV out."

—from Bill's diary

Dr. Lohmann stood looking at my arm and at the chart. "Where's her IV?" he asked the nurse.

She seemed to hedge a little. "I believe it was removed last night." Dr. Lohmann's usually expressionless face tensed visibly as he scanned my chart. "We'll have to check on this."

Here we go again. Why are these men fighting their wars across my bed? We already had duplicate X rays and blood work, plus the routine blood-gas tests. Most of these procedures started at five in the morning. The battle of clashing egos seemed to rage on. I tried to explain to Bill the conflict over the IV.

"I know." He let out a long sigh. "I talked to Dr. Lohmann. He says the pneumonia is eighty percent gone, but you still need the antibiotics. He said he's going to inquire about the IV." I saw my own agonized frustration in Bill's expression. "Don't worry, Sue. I'll get this thing straightened out." How, Bill? There is no way to "straighten out" this conflict. But telling that to Bill was pointless. He knew it all too well.

The next day the IV was reinserted. I knew it was necessary, but I could hardly bear it—one more symbol of setback. When Bill came in, his eyes were fixed on the IV, tears rolling down his cheeks. How can you keep coming here, Bill? This is just too much of a burden for you to carry. And why do I lay more on you?

No longer could I stifle the depression. I was going backward. Nothing more was being said about my moving upstairs. I didn't know what was going on and no one else seemed to know what was happening. I was being weaned a little each day from the respirator, but it was not going well.

"Hang on, Sue. This can't last much longer." Bill tried to encourage me, but could I believe that? I had to. It was all I had to cling to. Oh, Bill, how I love you. Without you. . . . I could not even think what would happen without Bill.

Suddenly, I remembered—Lissy was graduating from high school. Last year she and Bess had given Katherine a graduation party. Now it was time to do something for Lissy. I latched onto this distraction. Finally I had something to work on in these days of helplessness. Graduation was little more than a month away. We had to start planning on this.

Need to give Lissy luncheon for graduation.

Bill's eyes blinked, stared momentarily, and then rolled upward incredulously. I was not going to waste time and energy spelling an argument with him. I had it all planned.

Ask Liz make lunch reservations. Liz would know a good place to stage an appropriate luncheon.

Tell Elizabeth check Lissy on guest list. I could work with Elizabeth on getting invitations out. This little assignment for Bill was just to let him know I was back in gear again! He shook his head slowly in disbelief, and then the glimmer that began in his eyes grew into a full smile. What a beautiful sight! The past few days had left no room for smiles. Yes, Bill Baier, we'll make it now.

"March 21: Sue asked how I was!"

—from Bill's diary

Kay came back! Her new job had not been what she had hoped. I was ecstatic to see her.

"Come here, Phil," Kay called. "Help me turn Sue." They laughed and chatted as they rolled me over. When my arm flopped down, the IV tube pulled out. I knew it was no problem, because I'd heard the nurses and doctors earlier that day say that the IV was due to come out. They'd decided to leave it in until a series of medications ran out—just as a precaution.

When Kay and Phil saw the loose IV, they were upset. "We have to get it back in," Kay said.

No, no, no. But they wouldn't look at me. They were too preoccupied with this problem.

"It's going to be rough getting it back in," Phil said. "I've never worked with her, but they say she hasn't any veins left."

"Well, we've got to do something. There'll be trouble tomorrow if this thing isn't back in."

No, no! I pleaded. Look at the chart. You'll see that it doesn't need to be in any longer. But Kay saw only my protestations, not my reasons.

"I'm sorry, Sue. It has to go back in."

Phil grabbed the needle and began searching for a vein. "There. That'll do it."

No! Wrong! I could see and feel that it was in wrong. By now I knew how a properly placed IV felt.

But they were both relieved to have it reinserted. Kay didn't look at me. She just placed the pillows carefully at my back, patted me on the hip, and said, "You're all right now, Sue. Sleep well."

By morning my arm ballooned. The IV solution had seeped under the skin. My morning nurse removed the IV. Dr. Lohmann ordered that the remainder of my medications be given by injection.

Finally I was back in the wheelchair. I tried to make myself see this as a step forward, but optimistic self-sermons gave way to self-pity, to reality. Desolately I watched as the other patients turned on their call lights and nurses rushed to their bedsides. But no one asked if I needed anything. I had become fused into the inanimateness of that huge wooden chair that held me.

Bill pushed the doctors for answers, trying to find someone with a plan we could rely on and attempting to remedy what he could now see was thoughtless care. As he pushed, they— whoever *they* were; he didn't tell me that—suggested it might be time for a change. Perhaps I would be happier at one of the specialty rehabilitation hospitals.

No. No changes. All new staff. Can't do it.

In spite of all the problems, there were some people here I knew I could trust. Even the ups and downs here felt safer than the idea of an all-new environment. Moving was impossible. Gary assured us his department could do anything for me that any other facility could do. All I wanted was a room upstairs— and a chance to be a normal patient.

I felt greasy and unkempt, especially when I sat in the wheelchair and other patients' visitors walked past me. My hair hadn't been shampooed for days—there had been too many other things to worry about. Now Dr. Birmingham walked toward my bed. As I fought off my instinctive anxiety, he walked up to me and studied me. *What is he going to do now?*

"You need to fix yourself up. You remind me of my dogs when they come in out of the rain." I was devastated, even breathless for a moment. I'd heard the staff grumble about his abruptness, his temper that lashed out at whoever was convenient, and his tactlessness. In fact, I'd watched people disappear when he walked into the unit. I had been the victim of his rough actions, but this was the first time he had ever spoken to me like this.

Surely my eyes flashed the mixture of anger and hurt I felt. *Fix myself up? What do you think I can do about this?*

Still unbelieving when Bill arrived, I spelled out the insult to him. Always the conciliator, Bill tried to placate me. "Sue, I'm sure he just meant that it would make you feel better if you looked nicer."

His dogs are sheepdogs! Bill didn't laugh, but I knew he wanted to. "Sue, he's concerned about you. He didn't mean that. Don't let him upset you." The subject was changed quickly.

But I could not repress the thought of how dreadful I must look. I'd always had my hair cut every three or four weeks. Because my hair is very fine and thin, I've always kept it short and washed it every day. Now my long, greasy hair troubled Mother—I could tell by her gasp of excitement every time I had a fresh shampoo. But to have my appearance flaunted so crudely to me was unbelievably cruel.

"March 24: Get Lohmann and Birmingham together to stop duplicate X rays and blood tests."
—*from Bill's diary*

The battle waged on—and the duplications. My primary veins had virtually collapsed, and there was only one person in the hospital who could find the one remaining usable vein in my right arm. When she was not on duty or otherwise available, the rest of the technicians simply butchered me.

Bill finally had a long talk with Dr. Birmingham and discovered his role in my case! Since the director of respiratory therapy was not a physician, Dr. Birmingham was on call for that department in ICU. He had been called in for consultation when I was placed on the respirator and had stayed on the case.

Now Bill received a new promise from Dr. Birmingham: in one month I would be put into intermediate care. I'd be out of ICU and upstairs in a regular room. Could I believe that? Bill seemed to. This was different from all of Dr. Birmingham's other predictions. A month seemed so far away, yet I knew I could handle that, a definite date. If only I could be absolutely certain.

But his promise was all there was. I had no choice but to accept the thirty-day countdown.

15

Elizabeth announced her decision to run for Student Council office. This year had gone well for her. She was inducted into the National Honor Society and she and a friend were designated joint delegates to Girls' State from Lee High School. Also, she would be a section editor for the school newspaper next year. The election would be a good experience. But she hadn't decided which office to shoot for.

Her friends were encouraging her to run for president. "I couldn't get elected president, Mother," she said. I wasn't so sure, but Elizabeth was a pragmatist.

"Vice president. Perhaps I'd have a better chance at that," she decided. "Besides, I am involved in too many activities already to take on the presidency."

I remembered well the excitement of election time at Lee. Posters, slogans, fliers, various gimmicks. It was always a full-blown campaign. I wished I could be there again at my volunteer's desk, absorbing it all.

Elizabeth showed me her posters, discussed her strategy, and checked on what she should wear for her campaign speeches. We decided on an appropriate dress. When the time came, Bess and her tape recorder captured it all for me. Elizabeth talked about what she would do during her term. She concluded with, "And I'll show you who I'll be most concerned about during the coming year." With that, she lifted a Polaroid camera and clicked a picture of her audience! Bess told me the students reacted excitedly.

She won the office of vice president.

March was wearing to an end. Outside, spring was in full bloom. But in Bed Number Ten, life was sad, frightening, exhausting, frustrating, and boring—as it had been for seventeen weeks.

Mentally I erased the dragging days, first one, then the next, and a third—days that would take me closer to the promised move upstairs. Could I believe Dr. Birmingham this time? It had been three weeks since I was first taken off the respirator, when my hopes of getting away from ICU had been so high—three long, heartbreaking weeks. Now I desperately needed some small hope to cling to. A month was at least measurable. So I counted. And I shared my misery with Bill, who listened patiently day after day.

Morale low. Need TLC.

Again Bill bore the brunt. He wrote my words, put away his diary, and caressed my hand. The burden was all the worse for him because finally he understood the personnel conflicts that surrounded me, yet we both knew he was powerless to change anything.

On March 30, President Ronald Reagan was shot. Ginnie ran to my wheelchair. "Sue, the president's been shot. Let's put on your television." All the staff rushed in to watch.

As I stared at the screen, waiting for each news bulletin, I was immersed in the horror. When his surgery was finished, a hospital spokesperson announced that the president was in intensive care. I looked around the unit. It was not right that he should be reduced to this. I prayed for him.

During his evening visit, Bill and I sat silently, absorbed in the tiny screen. The word was that the president would recover completely, but Press Secretary Jim Brady was critical. A bullet had torn through his brain. There was some question whether he would survive. On into the evening I watched. Experts were interviewed. The president would have no long-lasting effects, they said, but Jim Brady was likely to be paralyzed the rest of his life—if he made it at all. Photographers caught glimpses of family and friends arriving at the hospital. I prayed for them all. Theirs was to be a long vigil—like the many long nights and days for my family. Such insanity! So much suffering. Hang in there, Jim Brady. We both have battles to win.

Eating became increasingly important to me as I drew closer to getting real food. The setback had postponed that pleasure, too—but not my new craving for food. For seventeen weeks I'd subsisted on IVs and the thick liquid diet forced down my NG tube. I wasn't really bothered by talk of recipes for the girls' party or the family's meals, or those frequently shared by staff in conversation, but it was hard to watch the nurses eating in the station. I could see them every shift, every day. Sometimes they'd phone out and order sandwiches from a deli—huge, plump sandwiches. When they felt talkative, they'd lean over the bed while eating all manner of food. And I'd want just a taste.

One day, Bess asked Bruce, "Isn't that terribly difficult for Sue, having to watch you eat?"

He just shrugged. "Oh, she's used to that."

I wasn't. It had bothered me from the beginning, but it was much worse now that I was in limbo, waiting for my recovery to get back on track. I watched with envy as the other patients received their trays and ate real food.

Often some asked, "Sue, what do you want to eat first?" I'd spell lobster or shrimp—and then lie there thinking about the tastes of different foods. I'm not a big eater, but now I was obsessed. I pictured myself in my own kitchen, picking out a recipe, gathering the ingredients, preparing a meal, and then sitting down with Bill to eat it. Or with the whole family. Or even with friends at a dinner party.

When Dr. Lohmann finally stopped the antibiotics, he had the dietitian stop in to see me. I would start with a liquid diet, Mrs. Reeve told me. No lobster or shrimp, but I would have the taste of food!

When a tray arrived for me and was put on my table, I had no idea what liquids might be under those warming covers. I waited and signaled, but no one came to feed me. All around me were patients eating or being fed their dinners. I wanted my dinner, too. When it was time to collect the trays, mine was hauled away unceremoniously—untouched. Trays came and went for days. A nurse would even bring the tube feeding while my liquid meal sat on my table. Then it was sent back with a wave as the feeding was forced down my tube. They apparently didn't have time for both. I kept hoping Dr. Lohmann would ask about my food intake, but he didn't.

"April 1: Birmingham says Sue had a good night."
                                        —*from Bill's diary*

I was astonished when Bill expressed pleasure at the report that I'd finally had a good night's sleep.

No! New nurse. Suppository didn't work for sleep.

How could Dr. Birmingham report that when, in fact, I'd had a terrible night and barely any sleep? Is that what was on my chart? Once again I saw the look of doubt in Bill's eyes. Who was he to believe? Did he feel, perhaps, that my depression was turning to paranoia?

Was I paranoid to want to be treated as human? To be asked how I felt? Did you sleep well, Sue? Are you comfortable? What would you like? We're sorry you must endure this rotten existence. There were so many little things, constantly, one after the other—indignities that led to my desperation.

Once again, the hours in the chair increased. Two and a half hours of uninterrupted agony. When a healthy person sits, there is a continual shifting of weight, movement from one side to the other, crossing of legs, little things to ensure comfort. But there was no way to shift and alleviate my torture. I thought about people who spent their lives in wheelchairs. How do they endure the discomfort? I tried to think about others, but the pain of my hips and tailbone was too acute to allow distraction.

I also tried to ignore the fact that I'd begun coughing again. Bill could not ignore it, and we both cried our fears silently. If only I could get everything coughed up, perhaps it would all go away.

"April 2: Feeling of dread. Birmingham says more time in chair in ICU."
                                        —*from Bill's diary*

Elizabeth's seventeenth birthday was April 5, and I was despondent at not being able to do anything for the occasion. Bill and Mother brought her to see me that Sunday, before taking her out for lunch. She actually seemed older. She had had so much responsibility all winter, being such a help to her daddy.

I wanted the two of us to make her favorite birthday cake again, a castle cake with a drawbridge made of chocolate squares and turrets made with ice-cream cones. And I wanted to hold her in my arms and give her a happy birthday wish. Instead, she was hugging me. "I love you, Mother." I couldn't even tell her how much I appreciated all she was doing. I fought back the tears as I watched her leave. She wasn't my little girl any more. She had grown up too fast. Where had the years gone?

After a week or so, the staff began to notice my dinner trays. There was no time for them to feed me during the day, but evenings were less hectic, so some nurses tried to help me with the tray offerings. Bland as they were, they had some taste. Still, most of my trays were being sent back to the kitchen untouched. Today, however, Bill brought me the first ripe strawberry from our small patch. He proudly carried his little treasure and patiently fed me minuscule shreds of the delicious, juicy berry.

Now tonight, here was Craig. "You're going to have dinner tonight, Sue," he said. It was extraordinary to hear Craig say anything. He was always silent and quite mechanical about his procedures. Now he was going to feed me a meal? He raised the bed a little, put a towel across me, and patted it in place. Next he brought in several huge syringes, 1½ inches in diameter. He attached a small piece of plastic tubing to each of the syringes where the needle was supposed to be. Craig lifted the covers from the dishes, and we both studied the tray. I had graduated to a soft diet.

"Well, let's see what we have here," he said, picking up the menu. "Ah! Pork, mashed potatoes, and apple sauce." It sounded wonderful to me. "Well, let's have at it."

Everything had the consistency of baby food, but the colors were right—and it was food! He drew small portions of my feast into the syringes, one at a time, and dropped dabs of each onto the back of my tongue, spacing the foods properly with small amounts of iced tea. I was tasting food! Trying to get anything from a fork or spoon was impossible—none of my cheek or lip muscles were working yet, and my tongue barely moved—but this ingenious technique worked, and I was thrilled.

"I often feed my little nieces and nephews," he told me. "It's great fun." And he now seemed to enjoy helping me. Throughout the rest of the evening, he got most of the dinner into me. From time to time, he'd leave to care for another patient and then come back to continue. I loved every "bite." It was my first real meal, and Craig taught me a technique I would teach my new nurses for months to come.

No one had time or inclination to feed me during the next three days. Again Mrs. Reeve came to see me. I suspected she thought the return of my full trays meant I didn't like what the kitchen was sending. She wondered what foods I liked. That was easy, but what could I swallow? One thing I was sure could go down was tomato aspic. Bill passed the word on to Mrs. Reeve and she assured him that if I wanted it, I'd get it. The aspic was delicious, but taste was about all I got. My swallowing was so slow that only the tiniest morsels could slide down my throat. No one could possibly have the time to feed me a full serving of anything. My main sustenance would continue to be the tube feedings, which were still stuffed down during every shift.

One afternoon, James arrived with triumphant fanfare, carrying a magnificent chocolate pie. This was not just a pie—it was a masterpiece.

"Dick made this just for you." I was overwhelmed. James and I frequently talked and spelled about his housemate's culinary exploits, but I never imagined something like this.

"We decided that we had to give you something you couldn't resist, so you'd eat more," he said. "You can start on this when Bill gets here." I laughed to myself; it would take me a month to eat all that pie.

When Bill arrived, James made another elaborate presentation. Then he cut an enormous piece for Bill to feed me and marched off with the rest.

"Now listen, everybody," James announced. "We're putting this in the refrigerator for Sue. This is her pie, so y'all keep your hands off, understand?" It was terrific to watch Bill laughing out loud!

He scooped up a few tiny spoonfuls for me to eat. I savored the taste of chocolate, but the texture made it too difficult to swallow. I could down only a few smidgens.

Eat, please. Don't want James think I didn't like!

Bill had difficulty pretending reluctance. The rest of the piece disappeared quickly.

One by one, the staff came by to drop hints about tasting the gorgeous pie. Soon there was begging and pleading. I didn't want to give the go-ahead, for fear of hurting James's feelings, but finally he himself asked, "Sue, can they eat it?"

Yes. It needed to be eaten. All that mattered was knowing it was mine. Nothing could dim the gratitude I felt toward James and Dick for this thoughtful gift.

Elizabeth and I were involved in serious discussions about Lissy's graduation party. We considered various locations for a luncheon, or possibly a Coke party at home. Elizabeth could handle that easily. Thoughts of luncheons, menus, and decorations continued when I was alone. Party planning seemed to be one of my most effective tranquilizers. Then one day I remembered that Douglas, Liz's son, also was graduating this year. As soon as Bill arrived, he heard the news.

Must give Douglas party. Liz did for Katherine. Our turn.

"A party for a boy?" I was prepared for the response—and for the look of absolute chagrin on his face.

Yes. Ask him what he'd like. Maybe take date to dinner and theater.

Bill dutifully wrote my words in his book, hoping he wouldn't have to read what he'd written.

After several weeks I was totally off the respirator. Did I dare to hope that this time it was for good? Next, if I could only get rid of the tracheostomy tube—then I could talk again. But I mustn't allow myself to jump ahead to that hope.

Charles came in with a bigger-than-usual smile. "This is it, Sue. Today we go to therapy. Are you ready?" Going to therapy—going anywhere—sounded just fine.

Yes. But I immediately had second thoughts. I wanted to go, but I remembered all too well my previous brief trip out of ICU before my last setback. I had been in such pain from sitting in the chair that I was virtually oblivious to what should have been an exciting first. Gary Stiller came in while Mother was visiting me and announced he was taking me for a ride. He and Ginnie took Mother and me outside to a courtyard for my first breath of fresh air. But I was in such excruciating pain that I couldn't even think about what was happening, or enjoy the time outside. At least today I was starting out fresh from my bed. Perhaps that would help.

Just getting me in the chair was an ordeal—disconnecting the sensors and handling my tubes, in addition to moving my limp body. Charles was getting expert at that, but still I wondered what would happen if I needed the respirator. He chatted reassuringly and carefully swung me into the wheelchair. I was too excited to notice more than the first stab of pain as my bones hit the hard seat.

After I was positioned and strapped into place, and the catheter was hung on the wheelchair, he looked at me in mock seriousness. "We have to do something with your hair."

He got my brush, and then a rubber band from the nurses' station, and he began brushing my hair. His massive hands worked the hair back and into, of all things, a ponytail!

"There. That's much better." His head cocked to one side and he smiled in admiration of his handiwork.

I tried to imagine how I looked, picturing wisps of hair flying out at the sides of my face. Better not to think about it, Sue. One time, as Phil was turning me, he pulled the bedside table close. "Sue, don't you want to see yourself in the mirror? You don't know how much better you're looking now." He started lifting the tabletop to expose the mirror.

No. I closed my eyes and refused to look. I knew how I looked. I saw my image in the eyes of my visitors.

The air felt cool against my face as Charles pushed me out of the cubicle and past the nurses' station. Several of them called out pleasant good-byes. Mentally I waved my response. Once the doors sprung open, I was elated. Out in the main corridor, people seemed to know who I was. People I recognized, and many I didn't, called me by name.

"Well, Sue, I hope you realize what a celebrity you are here at the hospital." I could hear the teasing in Charles's voice, but he was right. And for these few minutes, I was enjoying it.

We pushed through a pair of double doors. JoAnn and Ginnie were waiting with big smiles. "Welcome to PT, Sue," they both greeted me. Then Gary came strolling casually out of his office sporting a magnificent pair of cowboy boots. "Glad to see you again, Sue." My increasing pain seemed dulled by the sincerity of all their welcomes.

Charles turned the chair and we entered a bright, cheerful room. A pair of large glass doors flanked either side of a long desk area. Vibrant wall hangings brought life to the soft green surroundings.

"Here we are, Sue. This is where we'll be working in just a few days." He swung my chair slowly around the room, pointing out various pieces of equipment. He stopped when we faced the immense, stainless-steel tank. "And that, Sue, is the Hubbard tank. As soon as you get rid of your trach, you'll be working in there." Imagine! A bath. Real water to soak in. I couldn't wait.

"But today you get by easy," Charles said as he pushed the wheelchair toward one of the glass doors and up to a padded workout table. "I'm just going to put you up on the table and let you lie there and look outdoors for a while. Would you like that?"

Yes! He really did understand the discomfort of this chair.

Gently, carefully, he lifted me onto the table and positioned me on my back, with my face turned toward the outside courtyard. It had to be the one where Gary had taken me. "I'll be right here in the area, Sue, so don't worry."

I wasn't worried, not about anything. I looked out into a plain, empty courtyard, and it was beautiful. I could see sun and blue sky and a bush blowing in the breeze. I lay watching the bush, the most beautiful green I'd seen in a long time.

I couldn't control my tears as Charles pushed me back through the doors of ICU. This was the image I remembered from that first awful night. A nurse standing next to the station started to smile—ready to welcome me back—but she saw my eyes and turned away, silently sharing my desolation. Bed Number Ten was waiting.

When he had me positioned back in bed, Charles smiled reassuringly. "Don't worry, Sue. It won't be long now."

Please be right, Charles. I just can't bear this much longer.

Now that I would be going to the physical therapy room, I needed underwear. One more thing for Bill to take care of— bringing in fresh panties every day and taking them home again to launder.

The roses were again in bloom, so every few days Bill brought me a fresh rose—in addition to the radio and television batteries, *TV Guide*, underwear, boxes of facial tissue . . . and asparagus.

Bill knew how I love fresh asparagus. Our patch cost him his annual crop of tomatoes. Every spring he would spend two or three days preparing the soil for tomato plants. Everything had to be just so—all the nutrients in the ground and each little mound spaced properly. Several years ago, he'd just completed the preparations when I came home with twelve asparagus roots given to me by another volunteer at school.

"What are we supposed to do with these?" Bill asked.

"We could go stick them in the bed," I offered.

Exasperated, but without responding, he led me out to the garden, where I planted one beneath each of his mounds.

The young roots, which were two years old, required another year to take hold and then one more season before the asparagus was edible. But finally we got our first batch, and Bill had to admit it is the best crop we can grow. With just a little fertilizing, it keeps coming back every year, and our patch yields enough for us to have asparagus every other night during the season.

Now Bill had cooked the fresh, tender tops, mashed them,

and brought them in to feed to me one morsel at a time. Such a treat and a special touch of home—of Bill.

Getting me in and out of therapy every day became a major procedure, making my daily schedule even tighter and more tiring. First there was the struggle to get on my underwear. The catheter bag had to be emptied and then the bag was slipped through one leg opening. Next my feet went through the openings and the garment was shimmied up my limp body and into place. Since I was off the respirator, I needed a breathing treatment before I could leave with Charles—one more schedule conflict that caused tension as, watching us falling behind, I anticipated friction.

As soon as Charles brought me back to ICU, I was transferred to the bed and the oxygen was reconnected to my trach. Then the underwear was removed, with the original tedious procedure reversed.

That's when I became aware of an agency nurse named Elaine, a young woman with reddish-blond hair and glasses. Her eyes showed she cared. She saw when something needed to be done and often stopped by to do little things for me or talk to me, even when I wasn't her patient.

If Elaine was on duty, when Charles brought me back from PT, she'd scoot over to my bedside and take care of the underwear-removal chore. I wondered if she might be available for private-duty nursing when—and if—I ever got upstairs! I gave her name to Bill.

"April 9: Dr. Lohmann says Sue can go upstairs Monday."
—from Bill's diary

I couldn't believe it when Bill told me! In four days, I'd be out of ICU. This was almost two weeks earlier than Dr. Birmingham had predicted. I didn't mind the error. I was ready to leave.

Dr. Lohmann told Bill I must have round-the-clock private-duty nurses.

Talk to James and Elaine and get names of good people. I felt they both understood me and would be able to suggest nurses who could communicate with me.

Bill's face did not reflect my excitement. He was concerned about something. I waited.

"Sue, don't forget that the insurance company might not pay for private nurses. If that happens, you can't get out of ICU until you can move again. That's it."

They have to pay, I demanded silently. They just have to pay, and I must make it happen. Since my father had been in the insurance business, I knew anything like this took letters from doctors to explain the situation.

Get Lohmann or Birmingham to write letter saying I cannot talk or move.

Bill nodded his agreement, but I knew he would, as always, count on nothing until it happened.

"April 10: Another IV in for another infection. Lohmann says just for a few days. Will look at the X ray on Monday. Back in chair instead of PT. Tiredness. Setback!"

—from Bill's diary

Charles's expression, when he saw the IV back in my arm, revealed his feelings. We'd been making such good progress in therapy, but now it was halted. And the IV was set in such a position that it restricted arm motion.

But Charles was determined to keep some motion going. He knew—we both knew—that any interruption in the therapy would cause stiffness and possible swelling in the arm and hand. As he pivoted the arm carefully in a broad circle, the needle fell out of my hand.

I could see how he felt. His shoulders slumped as he smiled sadly. "Oh, dear. Look what we've done."

Charles received strong warnings from the nurses not to move my arm again. He suggested that they use a detachable heparin lock so he could disconnect the IV tube and continue my range of motion, but no one would listen.

Dr. Lohmann ordered the IV removed several days later. Once again physical therapy was resumed in full force. And again I was exhausted all the time. Which was worse—the pain of the chair or the total fatigue of PT? At least PT was activity, and it was moving me closer to recovery.

For so many months I'd tried to find ways to reach some level of communication with every member of the staff. I hated to give up on anyone.

Gary came in occasionally to see me in bed or in therapy. He'd always talk to me but never spell with me. That shut me out, forcing my communication to filter through Bill or someone else. There were so many questions to ask of this man who had such authority over my life. After all, Gary had declared himself the one in charge of my case—and I now believed he was.

One day he and JoAnn were together in my cubicle. I decided to try a lateral attack and spelled to the nurse: *Ask Gary to spell with me.* When she conveyed my message, he got a funny little twinkle in his eye and said, "In a few days, Sue." Then he walked off.

After a few more visits and still he hadn't offered to spell, I began spelling to anyone who was with him—Ginnie, Charles, Dick, whoever . . . *Gary spell!*

He'd respond, "Oh, I'm running behind," or "I have a meeting today. We'll do it next time."

It got to the point that every time he came near me, I spelled with whoever was there. The letters would start: $S . . . p . . .$

He'd quickly cut in, "Not today, Sue." He always put me off with a sarcastic little smile, and his unwillingness to communicate bothered me. I couldn't understand it. I felt a connection with him beyond his position in PT. After all, it was Bess who introduced us. And I'd learned he was active in a Bible study group with people I knew, a group that was adopting me in their prayers every week. Yet when I needed to talk to him, he refused. I was troubled by that. Was this his little idiosyncrasy? Or had this become a challenge of wills for both of us?

The possibility of a breakthrough with Bruce was another challenge. There had to be a way to reach him.

I'd listened to staff talking to Bruce. He was from New York and he liked deli-style foods. One night he was at my bedside, chomping on a corned beef sandwich while James suctioned me. This was my chance to "say" something to Bruce, since James would take time to spell with me. Bless his heart, he probably did more spelling than any other staff member.

Tell Bruce Bill also from New York area.

Bruce stopped eating for a moment. "Oh, really?" He resumed eating, but at least he looked at me.

Bill also loves corned beef.

James repeated the message and this time Bruce put down the sandwich. Could he actually be self-conscious about his eating? He couldn't imagine how enticing that corned beef sandwich looked to me!

Thanks to James, this was almost a conversation with Bruce. The next night he talked to me while he worked with my tube feeding. A few nights later, he told me he was about to have nose surgery to correct a breathing problem.

"I'm really concerned. I've never been sick before. I've never hurt. The thought of it scares me a little."

Yes, I thought, and that's probably why you can't seem to relate to me. I wished him well, but I hoped this might help him understand nursing a little better.

When Bruce returned after the surgery, his nose was heavily bandaged. He let it be known to everyone that he was uncomfortable, and I was fascinated by his reaction to the discomfort. He was not identifying with his patients' pain, understanding how we were feeling—he was just preoccupied with his own pain.

He never spelled with me, though several times I had someone else spell a message to him. There were times when I thought I saw a change in him, but then. . . .

During my last days in ICU, something seemed to obsess Bruce again. When a patient is ready to have a catheter removed after long-term use, the tube is clamped periodically for short intervals to let pressure build up in the bladder and restimulate the muscles. But I wasn't ready to be taken off the catheter. No doctor had mentioned it. Yet that didn't matter. Suddenly, for no reason, and without orders, Bruce began coming to my bed, pulling back the covers, and clamping off my tube. Just as he had told me that first night in ICU, "Get used to this," now he was saying, "I'm going to do this so you'll get used to it and know how it's going to feel when they have to do it to you."

This went on for at least two weeks, and he was the only person who ever did it. Because there were no muscles yet to support my bladder, I felt considerable discomfort each time he did it. But even worse was the bewilderment and the anger. Why, Bruce, why?

So much for communication with some people.

"April 10: Depressed. Both of us. Muenkel guesses six months more with home visits. Recommends transfer to rehabilitation facility."

—from Bill's diary

Monday came and went. The IV dripped on, and I remained in ICU. A heaviness set in again and Bill and I sank deeper into our despair. He went about the motions of getting in touch with Elaine and a few other potential private-duty nurses, but we were afraid to hope.

Charles tried to prepare me for the eventual move. He wanted me to be realistic about my expectations.

"Sue, as anxious as you are to get upstairs, you have to remember that the floor nurses are not going to be able to relate to you. If you get really good private nurses, you'll be fine, but the chances of their all being good are very remote. And when you're alone with someone who is not an intensive care nurse, it's going to be you and that person against the world. It will be different. No monitors, no backup. This is a big step."

He was right, and I appreciated his concern for me, but

nothing he said could dampen my burning desire to get out of ICU and into a real room.

Dr. Lohmann finally wrote the much-awaited letter to the insurance company. He brought it in during his regular noon visit—and he actually spoke to me! "Here's the letter for Bill. I'll put it in the drawer for him."

"April 16: Took letter to insurance company. Approved private nurses!"

—from Bill's diary

Bill, along with Mrs. Farrell, the director of nursing, Gary, and Dr. Lohmann, had a long discussion over whether I needed a private room or a double. The round-the-clock nursing staff and all the equipment I required would make it very crowded with another patient in the room. But this decision, Bill was informed, was out of our hands. The three of them would decide what was necessary.

Late in the afternoon, word came. Tomorrow, April 17, I would move upstairs! We were both afraid to ask any further questions. Another mild infection had developed, but I was assured it wouldn't stall the move. A heparin lock was installed in my wrist to handle the antibiotics.

Dear God, please don't let me be disappointed again! Please don't let anything go wrong now—when I'm so close. Only God could have heard my silent prayer. And the next day my prayer was answered.

April 17. Good Friday. This year the Friday before Easter would indeed be good for me. It was Moving Day!

The hospital administration decided that my belongings would be moved during my afternoon PT, and then I would go straight up to my new room. We had no idea who I'd have for nurses. Mrs. Farrell recommended that we employ the agency that the hospital used, and the agency assured Bill that someone would be there and that my care would be well covered at all times.

When Bill arrived after lunch, he and Carol, my ICU nurse that shift, began taking down the cards from my curtain. It was happening! There was much discussion about which cards should go upstairs with me and which Bill would take home. The Valentines could go, we decided, and Easter cards, which were already pouring in, should stay.

In spite of all the horrid months in ICU, there were regrets and second thoughts as I looked around the unit for the last time. A cleaning woman who was mopping the floor across the unit wrung out her mop, looked over at me, and waved. Just yesterday as she worked in my area, she repeated what she often told me: "I'm glad to see you are getting better. I've been praying for you." She and the other cleaning staff had become my friends. Several of them always reached out and patted my hand or the side of the bed when they came into my cubicle. I mentally waved back to the woman with the mop.

Truly, many caring people had done so much for me, and I *was* getting out of there without bedsores. Certainly my general care had been satisfactory—lack of communication had been the overwhelming problem. Whatever lay ahead, things had to be better with private nurses. For a fleeting moment I thought of being alone with an Aurilla for eight hours. I pushed aside the thought. That just can't happen.

I was more than ready when Charles came to take me to therapy. As he rolled me out the door this last time, my departure was quite unheralded. No one even noticed.

3

COMING
BACK

16

"This is it, Sue. Room 219." As Charles turns the chair to face me into the room, my room, I see Mother and Bill waiting for me, smiling. Quickly I scan the room, and there is only one bed! All the rooms by the nurses' station were supposed to be doubles, but to my left, where the second bed should be, is a big red couch. Across from it stands a desk. Opposite the bed, double closet doors are decorated with my cards and pictures.

"Ho, ho!" Charles says. "What do we have here?" He walks over and pats the couch and then checks out the desk. I stare at Bill in happy amazement.

"I don't know, Sue," he says, shrugging and smiling broadly. "Looks like some little elves have been at work. All I know is this is a semiprivate room, just like the insurance company ordered." This is incredible; it's a palace!

I nearly burst with happiness as I notice the window next to the bed. Imagine, my own window! My gaze flits in disbelief from couch to desk and back to the window.

Majestically, Charles lifts me into the bed. I had been so excited and elated I scarcely noticed the hardness of the wheel-chair, but now the bed feels good. I survey my new estate with pleasure. Mother is still standing motionless, happy tears rolling down her cheeks. Bill—dear Bill—just beams.

The nurses in ICU wore colorfully printed uniforms, but now a nurse in a white uniform greets me. "Hello, Sue. I'm Marjean. I'm your nurse for this shift." She is a small, wiry, agile woman. Totally natural. No makeup, no pretensions. I feel secure with her the minute she touches me.

$H \ldots e \ldots l \ldots l \ldots o \ldots$. She catches each letter. Bill has already taught her how to spell with me, and she understands!

Bill points to the phone next to the bed. Fantastic! A tele-

211

phone, a link with the outside world. "How would you like to talk to Katherine?"

Yes!

It doesn't matter that I can't talk; I want to hear her voice. Still smiling, he dials the number. "Hello, Katherine. Guess what? We finally have your mother in her own room. She's here and wants to talk to you." He puts the phone to my ear.

"Hello, Mother. This is so exciting! How are you?"

Oh, I want to answer! I look up at Bill, and he takes back the receiver.

"Just a minute, Katherine, she's going to spell."

Fine. Just fine.

"Katherine, she says she's 'fine, just fine.' "

He holds the phone back to my ear. What a wonderful treat to hear Katherine's voice again, telling me about a lecture she's just attended.

Bill has errands to run, so he and Mother leave together. Now it is peacefully quiet. The clatter and voices of ICU are gone, and I am with a kind nurse who will stay here in the room with me. I feel no fear, only joy.

A technician arrives to draw blood. As he looks for a vein, Marjean stops him. "You don't need to do that." Her voice is firm and direct. "She has a heparin lock. Here, give me the syringe." She draws the blood easily through the lock, just the way it should be done.

I am awash in happy tears as Marjean positions me on my left side, facing the large window, the sunlight, and the blue sky. A billowy white cloud blankets me in peaceful sleep.

As my eyes open, I feel all smiles. This is not a dream. I am actually here, out of ICU! The setting sun bathes the room in a soft, warm red. Marjean is seated at the side of my bed. There is a twinkle in her eye as she points behind me. Carefully she rolls me over to my right side, and there is Bill, resting on the couch. My heart embraces him.

The floor nurses come in to greet us, offering their assistance for anything we need. During the days I'd spent at the hospital when Mother had been ill, I had seen instances of floor nurses resenting private-duty people and refusing to cooperate. I am thankful we can count on this staff to help.

"April 17: I spend night on the couch."
                                                            —from Bill's diary

Marjean has signed on to work a double shift this first day, three to eleven and then eleven until seven tomorrow morning. Even though she quickly adapts to my needs, Bill wants to be sure she can handle me alone all night and can operate the alarm clock—still my only signal when a nurse isn't looking at me. So, after watching the evening news together—another joy, a regular hospital color TV set—Bill settles in on the couch for the night.

For the first time in 4½ months, there is darkness at the foot of my bed. Only a nightlight and the streetlights from below shine in the room, and I welcome both. After all that time bathed in brightness, I feel apprehensive about total darkness. Marjean is sitting nearby, ready to respond to any need. And perhaps the sweetest thought of all is that just a few feet away, my husband lies on the sofa *in my room*. Tonight, finally, my little universe is quiet, snug, and secure.

It's a new day, a Saturday, and Bill does not have to go off to work. He instructs the new nurse at seven. Suddenly Charles's prediction becomes reality: not all private-duty nurses are good. Sandy's ability to spell with me is limited, as are some of her nursing skills—she can't, for example, suction me properly. Now that I am out of ICU, breathing treatments will be my only contact with respiratory therapy. James, Kay, and Peter work primarily in ICU, where most of the respirator patients are assigned, so these friends are not readily available to me. Suctioning is now the responsibility of my nurses, and Sandy cannot give me any relief.

This new day is such a letdown. I am grateful to be out of ICU, but it is scary being at the mercy of a single individual who doesn't know how to care for me.

Get Elaine, please!

"I'm trying to reach her, Sue, but so far I haven't succeeded." Oh, Bill, I wish I didn't have to be such a problem. It's always something, isn't it? But we have to get nurses I can rely on.

"I'm sorry, Sue," Marjean is saying, "I thought you were told." No, no one told me that Marjean would only work weekends. I had been so happy to see her when she came on at three today, especially after my frightening morning with Sandy. But now I learn she won't be back until next Saturday.

"I go to the university full time during the week. I'm getting my nursing degree." Her capable hands are suctioning me, then washing my face and combing my hair. "I can work one double shift most weekends, if that will help you." At least that is something to look forward to—if I can just make it through all next week.

As Bill and I watch Marjean finish her paperwork at eleven, Trish introduces herself and listens to Bill's instructions. Very soon we see what lies ahead: Trish seems unable to spell with me or suction me. Nor does she seem to understand the clock, in spite of Bill's detailed explanation. He lies down on the couch with a sigh of resignation, ready for an up-and-down night.

This morning, Easter Sunday, Sandy returns. Bill has gone home to shower and change clothes, and I am frightened. I feel isolated. Easter Sunday is not quite the joyous occasion I anticipated.

"April 20: Lohmann says more X rays. A little worse. Fluids in lower left lung. Needs draining. Will be difficult."

—from Bill's diary

Another holiday has passed, and the new week begins. Will it be better? My door springs open. What a surprise it is to see Kathleen, one of the nurses who gave me such special attention on Christmas morning.

Her smile is radiant as she welcomes me to the second floor. "I'll bet you're glad to be here. And how about this room? Isn't this something?" She breaks into another big smile.

"Do you remember seeing me on Christmas?"

Yes.

"But you probably didn't notice me the day you came in last December."

No.

"I saw you then and have been keeping track of you ever since." As she talks, she continues smiling and watching my eyes for reactions. "I was just filling in down in ICU on Christmas. We usually shut down this floor over the holidays." Her eyes twinkle. "That's not our busy season, you know. So several of us filled in around the hospital on Christmas Day. I drew ICU, and I got you."

Someday, Kathleen, I'll tell you what you meant to me that sad, lonely day.

I can now lift my elbow just a little, so engineer Bill has been working on something new for a signal to replace the alarm clock. When the private nurses go out for lunch or a smoke, I am apprehensive at being left alone. The alarm clock can't be heard out in the hall or at the nurses' station.

Finally Bill has a new creation, a very sensitive toggle switch that attaches to the bed's guardrail near my elbow and is wired into the hospital call button. With just a light touch of my elbow, the light goes on in my room, outside the door, and at the desk. The staff is impressed with Bill's wizardry. Apparently many patients have difficulty using the conventional call button.

Nurses say to patent call button.

Bill shakes his head slowly. "It's taking care of you, and that's all I'm interested in." And take care of me it does. I feel much more at ease now, even with nurses who are less than competent. If things get too bad, I know I can call the floor nurses.

Bill says he is still working on reaching Elaine, but his evasiveness tells me there is a complication. I am trying not to set my hopes too high. However, I do have a nurse I like a lot who will take me every afternoon during the week. Yvonne is tall, large boned, good looking, well groomed. She has the prettiest eyes and smile. On her first day she clicked right in and spelled immediately, and now the afternoons and evenings go smoothly. Once again I have hope.

"I didn't want to take this job," Yvonne says. That surprises me, because she is very good with me. "When the agency called me to take on someone who was completely paralyzed, I said, 'I can't do that.' Then they began telling me about you. And Sue, they knew how to get to me. They put me in a spot where I couldn't say no." I am certainly grateful that they did that to her. "I thought I'd just come until they found somebody else." She smiles broadly. "I guess I'm stuck now." I hope she can see the smile in my eyes.

I don't want to open my eyes, to face this day. My lung must be drained this morning. I was very apprehensive all night—filled with a sickening dread—even though everyone tried to be reassuring. Who will be my morning nurse today? How much will she be able to understand and communicate to the doctor for me? When I hear the door open, I open my eyes reluctantly, and there she is: Elaine! Tears pour in happy disbelief.

So happy. Can't believe you are here.

Her eyes fill with tears, too, but she smiles and clasps my hand. "I can't believe it either, Sue. The agency really had to talk to me. This is a shift I usually do not work. Yet here I am."

"I'm Dr. Rockne, and I'm a pulmonary specialist." He has a kind face and is speaking directly to me. That's a rarity for a doctor around here. He shows me the bronchoscope and explains what he will be doing.

"Now, Sue, any time it gets uncomfortable, I want you to signal. All right?"

Yes. Anyone who asks for my response is reassuring.

"All the way through, I'm going to explain everything I'm doing. Anything I see, I'm going to tell you." This is extraordinary!

Dr. Rockne's nurse appears and introduces herself. They are both comforting, and I try to be calm. With these two and Elaine here holding my hand, maybe I'll be all right. An injected relaxant and local anesthetic help ease my fears.

"You're lucky, Sue," Dr. Rockne says as he picks up the long tube. "Because you still have your trach, we can insert the bronchoscope down it, rather than down your throat." So far so good. Stay calm, Sue. It's going to be fine.

"Well, Sue, there is a bunch of fluid down there." His voice is too serious. I don't want to hear any more. He holds the bronchoscope up to my eyes so I can see for myself, and that helps to distract my fears. I can actually see the mass as he describes it to me.

"We have to draw it out, Sue."

The long needle slides into my side. It hurts, but I don't signal him to stop. I want it to be over, and I trust Dr. Rockne. Elaine squeezes my hand, and I keep my gaze riveted on her until I feel the invader gone from my chest.

"It's over, Sue," Dr. Rockne says. His voice is kind. "You'll start feeling much better now." I believe him. "We'll give you something to let you sleep for a while." Sleep will be welcome.

But just as the grogginess sets in, Elizabeth and her friend Jane appear at the side of my bed.

"Hi, Mrs. Baier." Jane gives me a big hug. "It's good to see you again." She is completely unfazed by the sight of me. "I'm sure glad you're doing so well."

Jane's mother, Mary, has been coming to visit faithfully, but I haven't seen Jane since before Thanksgiving. And now, in spite of how I look, dangling NG tube and all, she is acting as if everything is perfectly normal. I have watched so many visitors react with shock, even revulsion. How can Jane handle this with such ease and naturalness? But I shouldn't be surprised—this is the way she is. She and Elizabeth chatter good-naturedly. Their easy banter keeps me included, even as I fight sleep.

Jane has a special fondness for rainbows, and she unrolls a large rainbow poster. While I struggle to keep my eyes focused, she and Elizabeth happily tape it to the closet door. After we admire the poster and their efforts to position it properly, Jane announces, "Well, we'd better go, Elizabeth." She gives me another hug. "Mrs. Baier, we'll be back." Next, my hug from Elizabeth. As the door closes behind them, I succumb to sleep.

Elaine and I didn't know each other long in ICU, so we have much to learn about one another. As she bathes me, she begins talking about my appearance.

"I'm going to bring tweezers. We have to pluck your eyebrows." Terrific! "We'll have to do something about your hair. Do you have a hair dryer?"

Yes.

"We must have Bill bring it. How about hot rollers?" I don't believe this! I felt totally grimy during all those months with little personal grooming, and now someone is talking about doing the things I've always done for myself. Elaine can read in my eyes that I am smiling all over.

Knowing that Elaine will be with me every weekday and Yvonne will come in the afternoons, I feel warm and contented. Overnights might be a problem yet, but then I am supposed to be asleep. Everything is going to work out. For the moment, I can relax.

Elaine is working on new, ingenious methods of handling my personal care. She discovers that the suctioning machine, which is still used regularly for my tracheostomy, will also work for draining the water after my hair is washed. Next she goes to work on my complexion.

"You're all broken out. What do you use on your skin? We have to get your face cleared up." I can imagine how badly the oils have clogged my pores.

"I'll bring some facial scrubbers tomorrow," she announces, "and whatever else it'll take. We may have to make you break out more before we get you cleaned up, but we are going to get your skin back in shape."

Hooray!

Charles has always put me into the wheelchair and taken me to therapy. Now Elaine can do this, and she stays with me through the morning therapy session. This is especially reassuring, because I am not alone when Charles lets me rest while he works with other patients. Each time that Elaine pushes me down the corridor out of the therapy department, I again feel the relief of not having to go back to ICU.

Our daily routine has developed quickly. I welcome the orderliness. At seven, when Elaine comes on duty, we take care of my medications and breakfast. They still have to go down the tube, but Elaine always tries to feed me a little off the tray, too. Next, she scrubs my teeth thoroughly and even uses dental floss. Then she washes my face and hands before we go to PT.

Charles continues to come into my room every morning with his cup of coffee and cheery greeting. I can see almost immediately that this annoys Elaine. She has established this room as her turf, and he is invading it. "Now, you're coming down to PT at ten today, right?" he asks. The question is nearly always the same.

Yes.

"Yes, Charles," Elaine also responds, very politely. For the first few days, she never speaks of his morning visits, though I can sense the irritation. Finally, it comes out.

"We're going down to therapy," she grouses, "and still he comes in here every morning!" For now, I can only spell to her that he needs to see how I am to plan my therapy for the day. When I can talk again, I will tell Elaine how Charles and his cup of coffee lifted my spirits during the long months in ICU with so little to keep me going. I smile to myself, happily knowing he will never stop these special little visits. I don't want him to stop.

After therapy and before lunch, Elaine bathes me and washes my hair. When she is finished, I feel clean! During my bath she turns on the television so we can both watch "Hour Magazine."

"You've been so cooped up, Sue. You need this distraction—a chance to see what's going on in the world." I never watched daytime television at home, and in ICU the TV set had to be stashed out of the way during the day. I like this exposure to what is happening in the outside world.

After my bath comes lunch, and that takes forever! Elaine tries to give me as much as possible from my tray, to force the mouth and throat muscles to work, but it is agonizingly slow. While I am eating, Charles often stops in again to check on me.

"How are you doing, Sue?"

Fine.

"Are you going to be ready for therapy this afternoon?"

Yes.

He looks over my tray. "Hmm, what have we here? Chicken soup. How nice. That custard looks good." I can feel Elaine tense as soon as he walks in the room.

Yesterday he came in at the end of my bath and my hair was in rollers. I knew it was frivolous, and the curl would fall out of my terribly fine hair as soon as I had the strenuous workout of afternoon therapy. But the curl does make me feel a little more feminine for a few minutes. I need that after being dehumanized for such a long time. I know I blushed, though, when Charles broke into laughter. Elaine bristled. I reminded her that men always laugh at women's beauty rituals.

Yvonne is right on time: three o'clock. Even before I see her, I always hear her coming to meet us in therapy. Every day she wears a taffeta petticoat that rustles when she walks. When I hear that rustle coming down the hallway, I can relax. I know Yvonne will be with me for the evening.

Elaine and Yvonne leave for about fifteen minutes to do reports and charting at the nursing station near my room. After that, I am in Yvonne's hands.

For the first few days, Charles put me back in bed right after we returned from therapy; now he makes me stay in the wheelchair until he leaves the hospital for the day. Even though Yvonne freshens me as soon as we get back to my room, I never feel that I'm finished with therapy until I am back in my bed. I'm so exhausted from the exertion and the discomfort of that miserable chair that I welcome a few minutes of rest.

About five-thirty, Bill comes, and Yvonne goes to dinner. This gives her a break, and Bill and I have a little relaxed, end-of-day time with each other. Our morning and noon schedules allow only brief time together, so we cherish this special half hour.

My dinner comes now, but I am never hungry this early, since lunch takes forever. Yvonne will warm the dinner in a microwave later.

Bill always checks the tray. "Hmmm, what do you have?" The question is purely conversational. The soft foods all look alike, and there are few surprises. I am so limited in what I can swallow that we always know what is coming.

Because eating is slow, my real nourishment still must go down the tube after I am too tired to swallow anything more. I try to stretch myself, increasing my food consumption to become less dependent on the tube, so meals continue all evening long, with short interruptions for visitors.

Yvonne keeps reminding me, "Sue, the sooner you can take more nourishment off the tray, the sooner that tube can come out of your nose." That is good motivation. But no one knows how much energy it takes to eat, concentrating on every muscle to chew and then to swallow without choking. What appears to friends and staff as relaxed evenings are absolutely exhausting.

The two unfailing bright moments of the evening are Bill's phone calls. First there is the early call to say, "I got home OK," along with perhaps news of Elizabeth's schedule for the evening—especially the name of the person who is driving if she is going out.

Then about ten, another call comes, this one the most precious of all. Whenever Bill traveled on business over the years, I could always count on that reassuring call every night. I cherish it especially now after all those barren nights in ICU.

"Good night, Sue. I love you."

I whisper silently, I love you, too. These moments of my life, at least, are returning to normal.

As parts of my body begin to move, Charles gives me exercises to work on at night. About nine-thirty, Yvonne and I begin these, which are finished by the time of Bill's second phone call. Finally, Yvonne writes her report for the next nurse and gets me ready for the night by washing my face, giving my skin an astringent treatment, flushing my catheter, and brushing my teeth and then my hair. It is our nightly ritual. As much as possible, I try to get the weekend nurses to follow the same procedure. I like living with an organized, orderly structure, and this is beginning to be somewhat possible.

Except for two scheduled turns, I usually sleep through the night.

Through these first honeymoon days in Room 219, I am nagged by one fear.

What will we do about no-shows?

Bill's face indicates he's been thinking about that, too. This can be a problem with private-duty nurses. An illness, perhaps, or a car that won't start. If someone doesn't show up for a shift, the previous nurse still has to go home, and the floor nurses don't know what to do with me or how to communicate.

Bill makes a point of being at the hospital before seven o'clock for his morning visit, just to be sure someone comes. Today no one came. The agency is apologetic, but that doesn't solve the problem, so my nurse this morning is Bill Baier. He is amazing. He has watched my care for five months, so I spell to him what to do, and he is very proficient. Fortunately Yvonne arrives a little early—Bill looks exhausted by then.

The afternoon nurses usually know earlier in the day if they can't make it, and they call the agency in time for them to find a substitute. But I shudder to think what would have happened if Bill had not been here this morning.

I always enjoy the weekends when Marjean works, especially when she is with me Sunday mornings. She turns on the television and we watch the First Methodist Church services. Marjean sings along with the congregation, while I join in mentally. This is a very special time for both of us, worshiping together.

Little by little, we are finding night nurses and backup nurses for weekends and days when Elaine and Yvonne cannot come. But always there is an uneasiness about potential no-shows.

Last night the agency sent a new, bright, bubbly nurse. As he does whenever we get a new nurse, Bill waited to check her out and train her. She walked directly to my bed and handed me a small card that read, "Hi, Sue, I'm Patti." Then she turned to Bill and handed him a card. His smile made me curious. After a few minutes of instruction from Bill, Patti took over easily, and Bill left.

Bill is here early this morning. As Patti goes to the nurses' station with Elaine, he asks, "Did it go all right last night?"

Patti fit in immediately, learning to spell and wanting to know everything I needed to make me happy and comfortable. She also was very chatty about herself and her interests. She loves sailing but doesn't own a boat, so she frequently serves as crew for people who do. She doesn't want to work full time, but she assured me she'd fill in on short notice when someone else can't make it.

Yes. She is very good.

"I thought so." He is smiling as he hands me the card Patti gave him last night. On it is printed: Expect a miracle!

"April 24: Birmingham wants more chair time. She needs change of gravity. He may close trach next week."
                                                    —from Bill's diary

Dr. Birmingham still drops in occasionally to see me, but now he enters my room with a great flourish. He swooshes in, kisses my hand, and gives me a hug—great show of affection. Why is he so affectionate? In fact, why is he coming to see me at all? Doesn't he know Dr. Lohmann is my doctor?

Elaine is despairing of my long and straggly hair. Elizabeth talked to my regular stylist, but he does not go to hospitals. Disappointing. What do we do now? Finally, Elaine remembers that Phil from ICU was a beautician before he became a nurse. Yes, he will do it—after lunch tomorrow. This means I'll be late for therapy, but even Charles agrees a haircut is a priority for me.

What a to-do is brewing. Just the thought of having my hair done is exciting! Phil arrives with scissors and a cape to cover me as I sit in the wheelchair. We decide on a short, simple cut. With much verbal exchange, the styling begins. Charles also comes up to help supervise. I listen to the comments as the scissors click near my ears, and hair flies everywhere. After Phil finishes, Elaine shampoos my hair and all three marvel at my new appearance.

"Now you have to see how nice you look," Charles announces.

Before I can protest, he swirls the chair around and I look into a mirror for the first time in five months. My breath stops. Shock! How thin I am! I've known I lost weight, but I never imagined the change. My face is gaunt, pulled on one side by wasted muscles, distorted. No wonder my visitors wore such startled expressions, no wonder some friends could not bear to look at me! The ugly NG tube hangs out of my left nostril, down to my chin, with a metal clip flashing at the end of it. I cringe with revulsion. Now I can understand why that tube has upset Mother so much. Nearly every day she has commented on it and told me how happy she will be when it is gone. I knew it was there, but I never saw it as an appendage to my face—so hideous.

The image in the mirror is thin, childlike. If I look so much better *now*, how must I have looked before? My skin is pale. There is no makeup to hide anything. My features look washed away. All my freckles have disappeared from the lack of sunlight. I try to lift a hand, wanting to touch my skin, but nothing moves. It doesn't matter; there is nothing left of the way I liked to look, the person that I remember.

"Doesn't your hair look great?" Elaine asks.

"You look terrific, Sue," Charles is saying.

Yes. The haircut isn't bad—a pixie cut. Mother will be happy. She has always liked that style on me. But my hair is dark. The sun bleaches my hair naturally—now it looks brown.

I hope no one can read my eyes. I must pretend to be as pleased as they all are, but that sight is so disheartening.

Sensing my sadness, Charles spins me around. "All right, Sue, we have to go to therapy. Enough of this foolishness."

As he takes me down the hall, he calls to all the nurses, "Look at Sue's hair. She's had a haircut." True to form, these dear people all make a big fuss over Sue's new look. They are so sincere, but I cannot erase the image in the mirror. Now I know how I really look.

I am right about Mother. She loves it. "Now if we can just get rid of that tube in your nose." I agree and resolve to force myself to eat more. I *will* get rid of it.

Bill grins broadly as he studies his transformed wife. "That looks better!" It probably does look better to him this evening, but I smile inside. I wore my hair like this back when I met Bill. Soon after our first date, I began letting it grow out, and Bill soon informed me that the new style was a definite improvement. When we looked at pictures from the company picnic I'd gone to with him and his sister, Bill said, "It's a good thing I liked you right away, because I didn't like that hair or the blouse you wore to the barbecue." I knew then that I was seeing someone with definite likes and dislikes, someone who would certainly let them be known.

Yvonne has finished my evening ritual, and I am lying in my bed, staring out into the darkness, fighting flashbacks of that face in the mirror. Suddenly the picture of Elizabeth's friend Jane dispels the melancholy. Dear Jane accepted me totally as I looked, seeming not to notice anything different about me. I was just Elizabeth's mother, a friend. The eyes of a child. . . . From her, perhaps, I can learn to accept myself.

"April 27: Virginia didn't show. Had to wait for Mary. It made me late getting to sleep. Mary will do four days."
—*from Bill's diary*

I've been upstairs ten days and am beginning to feel like a human being again, thanks to the attention I am receiving. But poor Bill is being worn to a nub lining up nurses for every shift, training each new nurse, and often sleeping overnight on the couch in my room.

"I'll call the agency," Elaine is saying as she picks up the phone. By now she knows either she or Bill should call Friday noon to see that I am covered for the weekend and to find out who will be coming.

As she listens, her smile says reliable people are scheduled. Bill will have a little free time over the weekend, and I have something to look forward to.

Visitors are coming more frequently now, and I am thrilled to see friends again. Mother's cousin Ed from Florida is coming in today. He has been like a brother to her, and our families were very close in my childhood. He and I always had a special relationship.

Mother wants me to look my best for him. "Sue, let Ed come while you're up in the chair," she suggested. "It would be so nice for you to be sitting up with us." I know my appearance bothers Mother, and to her I look more natural sitting up. I understand her request, but she doesn't realize I'd be in such pain in the chair that I couldn't enjoy Ed's visit.

I told them to come about four-thirty, knowing Charles will have me back in bed and I'll be freshened up by then.

Mother is noticeably disappointed when they arrive and find me in bed, but to Ed it is no problem. He sits down on one side of the bed, pointing Mother to the other, and begins to talk. They have not seen each other for some time, so they first cover the general family news, then begin on things they did in their childhood—escapades they pulled on Mother's brother and things he did to them. They exchange stories I've never heard. Such good therapy for me, seeing my mother so happy, having Ed here, and hearing all these wonderful stories.

Mother is still glowing over Ed's visit. She says she had forgotten many of those episodes they relived yesterday.

"And Ed said he had a wonderful time, too." A slight shadow

crosses her face. "But, honey, it would have been so nice to have you in the chair."

There is no way to explain, even if I could use words.

My scream is soundless; the pain is unbearable. Charles pushes repeatedly against my shoulder, trying to break loose the calcium deposit that has frozen the joint. Each time he pushes, the pain increases. At last he stops—for now. As he rolls me over on the workout table, I catch a glimpse of Mother's face. She turns away quickly and wipes her eyes with a tissue.

When I first moved upstairs, Bill explained to Mother that noon was no longer a good time for her to visit me—I desperately needed a few minutes' rest after morning therapy and my bath. Since Mother was curious about my PT, she asked Charles if she could come during my afternoon session. He agreed—as long as she promised to show no sign of distress at anything he did to me.

"You can't call out. You can't cry. If you can just sit there without any reaction, you may come." Mother agreed, and she began arriving during the last twenty or thirty minutes of the two-hour session—sitting quietly, watching and waiting for me to be finished.

Today she is not successful in her efforts to suppress a reaction.

I am thankful that Mother and Yvonne can talk together during our little trip back to the room, now also part of the daily routine. Yvonne has such a genial way with people that she breaks the tension after therapy and makes this a relaxed time for all of us.

Occasionally Mother gives me a manicure during her stay, and today she pulls the tools from her purse. Yvonne catches my look. Today I am too exhausted from therapy even to have my nails done. As Yvonne explains this, I see the shadow of hurt in Mother's face. After watching that particularly difficult therapy, perhaps she especially needs these few minutes of touching me, of feeling she can do something for me. But I am so drained. How could she understand anyone being too tired to be touched? As always, Yvonne smooths everything over tactfully, and the two of them chat pleasantly until Mother must leave. Yvonne has become my protector and advocate—and a diplomat of the first order.

"April 30: Birmingham wants to talk. . . . Birmingham off the case! Lohmann says trach out next week, maybe."
—from Bill's diary

17

"May 8: Infection. Possibly sinus."

—*from Bill's diary*

My room has become a greenhouse, alive with plants and flowers. As word got out that I was finally in my own room, the floral gifts began arriving—from friends and from acquaintances we scarcely know, from Bill's co-workers, and from people who know me from my various activities. Each new arrival means a great deal to me. However, to Bill they represent one more regular chore—the need to care for them. He is becoming a grudging green-thumber at home, grumbling about all the upkeep of house and garden plants, yet proudly reporting each one that starts to bloom. As with everything else, he now does what needs to be done to all the pots and vases in my room. I watch him, bemused, as he snips leaves and dead flowers, moving methodically from plant to bouquet to plant.

"This one's starting to look scrubby. What do I do?"

Cut back.

"Maybe it just needs more water."

No. Cut.

He clips a couple of inches off two of the longer stems and looks back at me.

More.

He proceeds to give the plant a proper trimming—and then waters it, just for good measure. The yellow leaves beg for mercy!

Mother is also assuming responsibility for the plants. The nurses love watching them both—Bill waters, and then three hours later, Mother waters. Sometimes the plants approach drowning!

"Happy Mother's Day, Sue." Bill is all smiles as he tears the wrapping off the gift he has ceremoniously presented. Laughter bounces through my body, tickling even my toes as Bill holds the gift aloft. A moisture meter for him to use on my plants! Another sensible Bill Baier gift. My plants will love it!

He takes down the Easter cards and hangs Mother's Day cards from him and the girls. All the other space is covered with get-well greetings, including the biweekly Snoopy cards that still come from George and his canine friend, Hure.

Once we established a schedule for my personal care, respiratory treatments, and physical therapy, I expected things to go on happily ever after. But this is a hospital, and nothing ever remains smooth.

My lunch feeding time takes longer as I eat more, and Charles grows impatient with the delays in my getting to therapy. Elaine is becoming more impatient with Charles's attempts to hurry the process. And I feel increasingly tense over the friction between them.

I now spend two hours each morning and afternoon in physical therapy. Charles starts every session with warmup exercises, followed by something very strenuous. Then I get a little rest period. Other patients come and go during the session; I see them all. Usually I am the first to arrive and always I am the last to leave.

We have graduated from range of motion for circulation to "the real thing." All muscle is gone, *all* of it. My arms and legs are mere bones covered with sagging skin hanging where muscle once had been. Charles and I must work to rebuild every muscle, which means getting the joints mobilized first. After all these months of paralysis, most of my skeleton is rigid. Calcium deposits, like the one Charles has been working on in my shoulder, have formed in joints all over my body, and all of them have to be broken loose for me to regain mobility. Breaking through each one produces excruciating pain. He pushes my limbs until they will move no farther. Then he pushes a little harder. Every move is done twenty times, each time going a tiny bit beyond the previous one.

I brace myself for one more shove of Charles's powerful grip against the unyielding shoulder. Finally the arm goes flat. A breakthrough! Our eyes meet and light up. The tiny grin that my static lips cannot contain reflects his joyful smile. Pain is forgotten for the moment. Charles calls in the rest of the department to see what Sue has accomplished. Time for a celebration. My nurses carry the good news upstairs and the floor nurses add their cheers.

There will be more celebrations, but in between, I know, will be days of frustration and increasing pain. There is no time for basking in any accomplishments. Always ahead lie more pain and more disability to conquer.

I try to keep my emotions in check during the agonies of therapy. I have always been a very private person. I don't often laugh out loud and I am very reserved in the way I handle my feelings. But as screaming pain continues, tears flow every day. I cannot hold them back. Charles also tries hard not to show his feelings, which are always close to the surface. He attempts to mask his own anguish, and when he knows he has to hurt me, he can't look me in the eyes.

"You know we have to do this, Sue. I'm sorry," he says so often.

Today was particularly difficult. Nothing moved. No celebrations. Charles was silent and seemed never to look at me through all that agony. Mother, Yvonne, and I are finally back in my room.

"I know it was bad today, Sue," Mother says sympathetically. "You couldn't see Charles's face, but I could. I thought he was going to cry with you."

Charles is talking today, as he does during most of our sessions—anything to distract me. He talks about his yard, the garden he is putting in. He tells me what he did over the weekend. He loves to cook and eat, and he enjoys talking about his gourmet creations. And always there is a new diet on the horizon.

We work so closely every day that I probably know as much about his private life as anyone else.

Other people from the department come in and out. Ginnie often works in the same room, frequently with hip patients. When someone new begins therapy sessions, she introduces him or her around the room, as if we were at a little party. This helps, since we are all in here together every day.

Sometimes, when I am about to wallow in self-pity, I am introduced to a new patient, a quadriplegic or someone who has lost a leg. I feel guilty for my own impatience as I see that the tiniest bit of new muscle has returned to my own limbs. It is coming back; I am getting well. And I am ready to work again!

A custodian, pushing a large cleaning bucket, stops at the door of the therapy room and smiles at me. "Charles, you're not hurting Sue today, are you?" he asks. He winks at me and moves on, not waiting for an answer. Everyone in the hospital seems to know how grueling and painful my therapy is, and they constantly are cheering me on.

Mobilization of my hands has become the most painful of all the treatments. No matter what else Charles does to me, this is the worst.

My fingers are straight and rigid, frozen close together. Each time he begins to work my hands, trying to bend the fingers, they grow red and puffy. My nurses soak them after each session and apply lotion, but still they look as painful as they are.

I stare at what were once long, slender fingers, and they do not even look like my own hands. And I still miss my wedding ring. Will these fingers ever bend?

Throughout these weeks of therapy, I have waited for the day I can get into the Hubbard tank. Charles mentions it often.

"Golly, Sue, as soon as that trach comes out, we're going to get you in the tank." His eyes sparkle with excitement. This is a big step, and it won't be long now. It is something positive to look forward to.

Sometimes, Charles pushes my chair over to the side of the

tank and says, "Here it is, Sue. We're going to fill it with nice, warm water and you're going to be in it in no time at all."

I can't wait to get into that huge stainless steel bathtub, down into the water. At home, I regularly took showers, but I loved to soak in a nice, hot tub a couple of times a week, just to relax. It seems like forever since I've known the soothing feeling of warm water.

"It won't be long, Sue," Charles promises.

"May 11: Charles stood Sue up!"
                                              —from Bill's diary

If Charles pulls me up into a sitting position and sets me at the edge of a therapy table, I can hang onto the table and sit alone.

We are at the end of the afternoon therapy session, and the look in Charles's eyes says we are going to play his little game: What can we get Sue to do today?

"Just one more thing, Sue," Charles says. His grin grows impish. "I think it's about time we stood you up." Stood me up? I can't do that.

The table is low enough as I sit that my feet are flat on the floor. Charles is standing in front of me. He puts my hands on his shoulders and places his large, strong hands on my sides.

"Hold on, Sue, and let's pull." I am excited, but not afraid. I am never afraid when Charles is holding onto me. Slowly, steadily, he stands me up in front of him. It is astounding, thrilling. Tears come immediately to my eyes, but I feel the smile pushing on my lips. He has me steadied, and a quizzical look appears on his face. Charles, who probably stands five-foot-eight or five-foot-nine, looks up into my eyes. "Sue, you *are* tall."

Ginnie and Yvonne are standing watching us, and both are laughing convulsively at the two of us standing there.

I am trembling, but still I feel no fear. I am secure.

It is only a minute or two before he eases me down again, but I have stood up for the first time! PT celebrates. Yvonne spreads the word upstairs, and soon all the floor nurses come in to congratulate me on my accomplishment. We are like family now. They often come in to see me, even when they aren't needed to help my nurses. But on these special days, they really help me celebrate.

I can hardly wait for Bill. He needs some good news, too. As I lie waiting, I laugh to myself, thinking about the expression on Charles's face as he looked at me standing in front of him and said, "Sue, you *are* tall." It has been some years since I have experienced that reaction.

I was always tall, just like my daddy. They called me "Daddy's *little* girl," but that was because I looked like him and I was tall like him. In all of my school pictures, right from the beginning, I was always in the back row, among the tallest students. By the time I entered high school, I was pushing five-foot-ten and still growing. I don't remember my height being much of a problem in high school, perhaps because I dated a boy who was a little taller than I.

In college, though, it was different. Friends were always trying to arrange blind dates for me, and I soon discovered that the rest of the world was much shorter. Girls would say, "Sue, he *is* tall." And when I'd meet the young man, either I looked him straight in the eye or I looked down at him. Or, at a dance, a fellow would approach where I was sitting and ask me to dance. Before I ever stood up, I knew what I was going to hear. "Oh, you are tall!"

In all these months of working with me and transferring me to the chair, workout tables, and bed, it had never registered with Charles that I was six feet tall.

"May 12: Trach tube out!"

—*from Bill's diary*

Charles has been anxious for the tracheostomy tube to come out. I want to get into that Hubbard tank, but I am also a little nervous at the thought of having the tube removed. I still need suctioning and breathing treatments. As much as I want to be rid of the trach, the idea of not having it is also scary to me.

Dr. Rockne, followed by Peter, has just strolled into my room.

Their expressions are suspicious.

"Here, let's have a look at that trach," Dr. Rockne says. As I study his eyes, I see a glint. All of a sudden, he reaches his hand up to the trach. Zip. It is out—just like that. I am astounded. It hurts only for an instant.

"There!" he says. "It's done."

Yvonne is laughing. "Sue, you can talk now. I can't wait to hear your voice."

"Wait just a minute," Peter says. "You have to talk to Charles first."

As Peter puts a gauze pad across the hole in my neck to allow my voice to activate, Yvonne is dialing Charles's extension. When he answers, she gives the phone to me. I can't think of anything to say; I am speechless. I was always very shy in school, and that's how I feel now: like a timid schoolgirl who has to speak before the class.

Peter and Yvonne are looking at me with obvious excitement. Charles's voice comes through with a tinge of impatience, "Hello." I don't even know if my voice will work. "Hello," he repeats—with a touch of annoyance.

"Hi, Charles," I say finally in a voice that sounds strange to me. I am so excited I don't think I am even moving my lips.

"Who is this?" he asks. Yvonne takes the phone and explains. Almost before she finishes, it seems, Charles is in my room, radiant—his whole face is one big smile. Word spreads throughout the hospital, and staff members from all over flock in— Ginnie, James, respiratory, floor nurses. Within minutes, the room is full. Everyone is crowding around the foot of my bed, laughing and clapping, wanting me to talk. I am so embarrassed at all the attention that I can't utter a word. I just lie there in shock—thrilled to death, but scared, mighty scared.

Charles assures me that the little hole in my throat will close up within a week or two, and then I can get into the tank. We're on our way.

Bill stands at the door for a minute, smiling.

"Hi, Bill." That sounds right—to both of us. We just grin and cry—and talk together all through the visit.

He is ready to leave now, and I know what I want to say, but again I feel shy, embarrassed—just like when we first went together. It hadn't taken me long back then to know I was in love with Bill Baier, but I couldn't tell him so. Even when we were engaged, the words still wouldn't come. It wasn't until shortly before our wedding that I finally knew I could say those words. From then on, they came easily—until tonight.

Bill is leaning over now to kiss me, and my overbrimming heart sends the "I love you" softly across my lips. Tears pour from both of us as he holds me in a long, warm embrace.

"Oh, Sue, I've waited so long to hear that. So long. . . ."

Tonight, when Bill phones, I am the one who says it first. "Good night, Bill. I love you."

Once Charles hears my voice, it becomes his goal to make me speak louder. Every time I speak, he yells at me, "Louder!" He just cannot understand that I have always been soft-spoken. He is determined that what I need is to exercise my lungs and vocal cords so that I can shout.

"Sue, speak up."

"But Charles, this is the way I talk."

Still he pushes for more. "Now, Sue, you must practice saying the alphabet and counting to ten, getting louder and louder." He moves farther away from me. "Now yell it to me."

Finally Bill explains, "Charles, Sue doesn't have a loud voice. It's not going to get much louder than it is right now." I think Charles believes Bill. After all, a husband knows how loud his wife can shout.

One thing I don't need to practice is talking. After being silenced for nearly six months, I can't stop talking—especially to Bill. It is wonderful to communicate all the little things I never had enough time or energy to say—to straighten out all the past misunderstandings when things were not as they appeared. There is so much catching-up to do.

Elaine could not make it to work this morning, so Bill took over at seven and stayed until noon. Now Katherine has come to relieve him—just in time to feed me lunch. I am excited to have her here, the first time I've been alone with her since she came home for the summer. Now we can talk. I don't want Charles to come in for PT. I don't want any visitors. This is my time alone with Katherine.

It is a difficult chore for her, feeding her mother. It's an awkward exercise, hard for her to know how much to put in my mouth at a time, or how my swallowing works. She is apprehensive, afraid I might choke. Being in Nashville, she was spared the day-to-day reality of my illness. Having my helplessness dumped on her now in such a massive dosage is almost too much. I am sorry it has to be this way, but I love having her with me for these few hours and hearing about her college experiences. It is certainly different from my days in college. Was it really a generation ago that I went through this? Katherine reminds me of myself in many ways—especially her determination about the choice of school. She chose Vanderbilt despite discouragement from Bill—just as I chose SMU a generation ago.

Somehow, my parents and I always assumed that I would go to college. In those days, not many of my high school classmates planned to go on to school. We lived in a farming community, and most of the boys went to work on the farms. Many of the girls would soon marry them. I didn't fit that mold, but there was a difference of opinion over *where* I would go to school. I wanted to go to Southern Methodist University in Dallas, because that was where Daddy had gone. My parents, however, felt that after a small high school, I needed a small college. And that's where they originally sent me, to Southwestern in Georgetown, Texas, outside of Austin. Some good friends of theirs had graduated from there and assured us it was a good Methodist school.

I guess my parents talked me into it, and by the time I left for Georgetown, I had decided that it was what I *should* do, even if it wasn't what I *wanted* to do. But once I started classes, there seemed to be nothing to do except study. There were none of the extracurricular activities I was accustomed to. Southwestern wasn't what I was looking for. I was determined to go to SMU the next semester.

My parents talked to the registrar at Southwestern, and she told them, "Let her go. That's where she wants to be, so that's where she'll do best." I was very happy when I got to SMU. There were about five thousand students, as well as everything I was looking for in both business and home economics classes—and plenty of outside activities.

After my own experience, I was pleased that Katherine stuck by her choice of schools. And now I'm happy she is finding what she wants at Vanderbilt.

Bill opens his briefcase and unpacks his lunch—a sandwich, a Twinkie, and an apple. While his after-work visits are still the longest and most relaxed, noon has also become special. His lunch is always the same, but at least he eats it with me. Because his visits in ICU were so short, he would inhale his food before or after his visit.

Elaine goes for her lunch while Bill is here. While he eats, I tell him the funny little things that have occurred to me. These private moments are especially precious after not having them for many long months.

No one has come to visit this noon, so after his lunch, Bill pulls up a chair beside the wheelchair, and we hold hands and doze—perhaps ten minutes. The warmth and comfort of these minutes seem to anesthetize my painful hips.

Sometimes Bill sets his watch alarm, but usually the nurse will awaken us when she returns and opens the door. It is rest we both need, and it is sweet to wake up with Bill holding my hand.

Now that I can talk, ICU nurses and respiratory therapists stop in frequently during their lunch or coffee breaks. It is fun to be able to converse with them. They seem to enjoy getting to know this person they never saw move or heard speak.

Ginnie's periodic visits to my room remind me of her little Sunday evening physical therapy sessions. She was so faithful all the while I was in ICU. Rarely did she miss, and when she knew she couldn't be there, she'd apologize and explain ahead of time. But it always seemed strange to me that no one ever took over for Ginnie when she couldn't come.

I decide to ask Charles about this.

"No one came, Sue, because no one is on the schedule for Sunday evenings."

"Then why did Ginnie have to come every week?"

"She didn't have to, Sue. She came because she wanted to come."

"I don't understand. Why did she work nearly every Sunday night?"

"She just came in to work with you because she couldn't stand to know you were lying there without any range of motion from Saturday morning until I got you on Monday." He resumes working on my fingers. "She and Rob used to come over this way to do their laundry so she could run in and out of the hospital and take care of you."

"You mean she didn't get paid for all those Sundays?"

Charles smiles, shaking his head slowly.

I am incredulous. She actually came in week after week just to take care of me? As I try to sort this out, Ginnie comes into the therapy room, all bright and cheerful. She looks at me, and as our eyes meet, I feel a flood of tears. I try to speak but can't. Words won't come. I just stammer silently.

"What's wrong, Sue? Is Charles being mean to you again?" she asks, laughing with mock sympathy.

"I told her, Ginnie," Charles says.

"Told her what?" she asks.

"About the Sunday nights."

Ginnie looks away. "Oh." No snappy, bright response this time. She hurries off to her patient. What an extraordinary gift. It will be months before the opportunity comes for me to thank her, and even then, words are inadequate.

"May 16: Sinus infection continues. Lots of phlegm. Needed suctioning through hole."

—*from Bill's diary*

Lissy's luncheon is on hold; her schedule at graduation time is so busy that we'll have to postpone it until later in the summer. Now, however, we must take care of Douglas. Bill is arranging for him to take a date to dinner and a performance of *The Student Prince* at Jones Hall.

"He also should have a small gift." Bill's sigh is expected. "After all, for a girl we would get some small keepsake. Douglas deserves as much." I settle on a silver bookmark; Elizabeth can select it. Bill arranges for the dinner bill and the theater tickets. I know Douglas will enjoy the evening, and so will I.

I wish I could be going to Douglas's and Lissy's graduation. I loved all that excitement last year with Katherine. Suddenly I am thankful I am sick now rather than next year, when Elizabeth will be graduating—if I have to be sick at all! After Elizabeth goes off to school, it won't be long before we start college commencements. I sigh and smile, thinking of my own college graduation. Someday, when the girls are finished with school, I will tell them about my graduation night at SMU.

All through college, I was about as straitlaced as anyone could be. With this "talent" for doing the correct thing, I was named monitor of my sorority house during my junior and senior years. It was my responsibility to check the girls' rooms—it's hard to believe they used to do that sort of thing in colleges—and if they didn't make their beds, pick up their clothes, or whatever, they received demerits and could be grounded or disciplined. They tried to tell me that I was the perfect one for that job because nobody got mad at me. But it embarrassed me to report anyone. I would wait around in the morning as long as I could, hoping everyone had time to get her room done. Terrible.

There was another girl in the house who also had a reputation for always doing the proper thing, and we both happened to stay at the house the night after graduation. That night, we decided we had to do something mischievous, break some rule before we left.

There's a fountain in front of the main hall at SMU, and students were strictly forbidden to step into it or put anything in it. So we walked out of the house, *after hours*, went to the fountain, took off our shoes, and walked around in the water.

We didn't get any particular pleasure out of doing it—no one even saw us—but at least we did have the satisfaction of breaking two rules before we left campus.

A new step forward, they tell me. I am being put on a portable commode every morning. It is about time for those muscles to start performing. I am very wobbly on this inauspicious chair, and the hard seat is painful. Sitting out in the open in my large room, with people coming and going, is hardly conducive to such a private function. Impatience is counterproductive, I know, but I want very much to regain control. So each day I endure the discomfort and humiliation for "just another minute"—and each time it is all in vain.

Most of the staff still refuses to believe that every minute is misery in the big, wooden wheelchair. After all, they are putting pillows under me. No, the real problem, they insist, is fear—I am fighting the chair because I am afraid of it, which is preposterous. I am afraid of the pain, not the chair.

Marjean, who formerly worked in an occupational therapy unit, tells Bill about a special cushion filled with gel. She is sure it will help me in the wheelchair, and I am anxious to try anything. "They advertise that you can sit on an egg on this cushion and not break the egg," she says. She advises Bill to check with a hospital supply rental company. "I'm sure you can rent them."

Several days later, Bill walks in at noon with a box. He lays it on the bed and looks at Elaine and then at me. A moment of silence.

After a deep sigh, he says, "This cost me $94. If it doesn't work, don't tell me!"

I try not to laugh. Elaine is startled and surprised. In the box is the pillow, complete with a plastic egg for effect. They do not rent the pillows, so Bill had to buy one.

Bill lifts me as Elaine slides the cushion under me. It squishes when I sit on it. Because I am so bruised, the new cushion can't alleviate my problems immediately, but it is more comfortable. I assure Bill that it is a big help. He chooses not to question me— just in case. We don't talk about the cushion any more today!

"May 19: 24 weeks. Feeling impact—running Elizabeth's errands, cooking, visiting. No end."

—from Bill's diary

Bill is growing very anxious for more progress. He wants me to be home as much as I want to be there. Now he has a new routine for his evening visit—a regular inspection of my progress as soon as he walks in the door.

"What moved today?" He is so full of anticipation that it hurts me when there is nothing new to report. He needs each high as much as I do.

He stands at the foot of the bed, leans down so his eyes are in line with my body, and checks over everything. "OK, let's see the toes move." I try my best. "Big toes move a little in both directions!"

A bit more of a smile with my mouth, an inch higher arm lift. If there is nothing new today, he reminds me of what moves now that didn't move a week ago. Bill never falters in his cheerleading.

18

"May 23: Saturday do-list. Weed side flower bed and asparagus bed. Fix banana plant. Fertilize roses. Put out snail bait. Drain lawn mower and put in new oil. Fix bicycle tire. Take laundry. Fix switch on electric toothbrush. Write thank-yous. Wind clock. Check air-conditioning system. Call Sue."

—*from Bill's diary*

The pendulum has swung. From the euphoria of having my own room and private nurses, I am sinking into the despair of having spent twenty-five weeks in the hospital, the grindingly slow return of my muscles, and the exhaustion of four hours a day of agonizing physical therapy.

Charles, once my supporter, my friend, has now become my taskmaster. His frustration that I am not progressing fast enough drives him to push ever harder. He's worked with only one other case of Guillain-Barré syndrome—a much milder case—and that patient was out of the hospital in three months. But I am not improving at the same rate, and this disturbs Charles. He seems convinced that if he and I work hard enough, we will get the job done faster.

On a workout mat he positions and twists me, struggling to pop calcium deposits or to loosen a frozen joint. It is awkward, painful, and frustrating. Most patients can be told, "Hold your leg like this," or "Bend your arm this way." But I don't have the control to do these things, and this taxes Charles's patience.

He is also frustrated because the trach hole in my throat is not closing, so I still can't go into the Hubbard tank. This is upsetting to me, too; I've waited a long time to feel that warm water. But to Charles it means continuing limitations on the therapy he can do without first limbering me up in hydrotherapy.

243

Nerves are fraying. Gary and Charles tell Bill I am deliberately spending too much time eating, trying to delay going to therapy. I plead with Bill to tell them I must eat, and it just will not go down any faster. Chewing and swallowing each morsel is tedious and time-consuming.

Now Gary stands beside my bed, hands in his pockets. "You have to stop this stalling, Sue," he says. "You're hurting yourself. Physical therapy is the most important part of your day. Now, from here on, this is the way it is going to be. . . ."

I calmly interrupt. "When I was a new patient in intensive care, you said you were pleased because Bill told you I'd always exercised." The words spill out. "I played tennis and I swam." I have his attention. "And you said, 'Sue, since you have made yourself do all these things that are good for you, you're going to be better off now.' This still applies. I am doing therapy now to help myself. I know that I am the one who is going to suffer if I don't."

He is backing down. "Well, we're doing all this for your own good."

"I'm very aware of that, but I also know what my body will and will not do, and I will push myself as hard as is humanly possible. However, I also know I must eat to gain weight and strength. And that, too, is for my own good."

He leaves, his hands still in his pockets.

Bill arrives soon afterward. "Well, Sue, I hear you and Gary are at it."

"What did he say?"

"Just that you aren't cooperating."

I can't believe this—Gary didn't listen. He is still blaming me for my slow recovery, and he is also trying to pull Bill into the middle of the conflict. This time, however, Bill knows I can speak for myself, so he'll just watch from the sidelines.

The cold war between PT and Sue Baier continues for several days. I feel the chill.

I question myself. Am I getting paranoid? Do I really need pushing from the staff? Do they have to make me mad enough to fight so I won't just give up and quit altogether? I can accept that much. Yes, I have to be pushed, and we must keep working. But I resent the accusation that I am deliberately delaying therapy. They are the professionals. They were supposed to anticipate all these things—the stages of my recovery as well as the importance of eating. But they can't—or won't—understand my position. What more can I do to reason with them?

Something more drastic has to be done about my stiff, straight fingers. They have to bend. Charles says there are devices that can be ordered, but he wants to try something else first. He sent Bill out to buy heavy gardening gloves and large safety pins. From now on, any time I am not in therapy, and especially during the night, he wants me to wear the gloves, with the fingers pinned to the palms to force the fingers down.

There is no way to describe the pain.

Bill finds me in tears, having had no sleep. Charles still believes I am not cooperating, so he is not being the kind, supportive friend I've come to trust. I need a little tender loving care, and Charles isn't giving me any. For the first time in all this illness, I cry out to Bill, "Why me?" Once again we shed our tears together.

"Why does Charles blow hot and cold? How do they know how much I can take?" Bill has no answers. He just listens and comforts me.

"May 30: Charles discouraged. Does what he thinks situation permits. Must push respiratory challenge. Much coughing, phlegm. Antihistamine every three hours. Trach hole shows moderate staph. Antibiotics."

—*from Bill's diary*

OK, Sue, I tell myself, we have to get along and make this therapy work. If I eat less breakfast, it will go faster, and my stomach may be less apt to get nauseous during therapy. I'll just have to make up the extra calories later in the day. The Sue Baier

who studied dietetics knows that breakfast is the most important meal of the day, so my decision troubles me. But we have to
get back on a smooth course with PT, and this is one way to
make it happen.

Is it my imagination, or is my stomach growling? At least
Charles is pleased to see me arrive on time for therapy.

There's that look again in Charles's eyes. What is he going to try
today? I am standing in front of him. My knees wobble, but I am
secure in his grip.

"OK, Sue, lift your foot and take a step." He sees my surprise.
"Come on. You can do it. I won't let you fall."

I concentrate on every muscle and joint in my left leg. Nothing
wants to move. Then, ever so slowly, the foot responds to my
commands. It takes a step!

"Now the other foot, Sue. Come on. Keep going. Just one
more!"

Again total concentration. I issue the message to my right
foot, again and again. Go. Go.

It shuffles forward the slightest bit. But it is a step!

"You did it, Sue; you did it!" His hands are trembling with
excitement, but still he holds me firmly. Both of us are crying.

"Sue, there are people in this hospital who said you'd never
move again, let alone walk. But they were wrong, just as I
always knew they were! You have just walked!" More smiles
and tears, and another celebration in PT.

The war is over between us. We are a team again. The whole
hospital rejoices with us.

Of all the cheers over my newest accomplishment, the most
touching is a card from Bill's father. He always had a special
talent with verse, and before his stroke, he wrote clever poetry
for every occasion. Bill still treasures the poem his dad wrote for
his graduation from high school, and I have saved the verses he
sent for birthdays and anniversaries. His beautiful handwriting
also enhanced each greeting. But it all stopped after his stroke—
his writing hand was paralyzed. All he could manage now was a

laborious, "Love, Dad" on a card or letter sent by Bill's mother. Since I've been ill, greetings have come often from Bill's mother, always with an encouraging message passed on from Dad.

Now comes a card addressed to me and signed with the labored words, "Keep up good work. Love, Dad." What a boost this is from someone who has suffered with me each day.

"June 5: Call Dad. Thanks for letter."
                                        —from Bill's diary

It is June, and we are moving again. Orders are to begin clamping the Foley catheter to distend the bladder. That is encouraging. And this time there is no discomfort; the bladder is ready.

Dr. Lohmann has come in for his daily visit. He speaks briefly with Elaine, and then I hear, "Let's take out the NG tube." Before I can fully register what he's said, he reaches over and takes hold of the tube, and out it comes. I am startled—and delighted. I want a mirror immediately, to see myself without that ugly appendage. This is better, a lot better. But the lack of facial muscles still bothers me.

Since that tube always disturbed Mother, I have been anxious for her to see me without it.

She has been sitting quietly, as usual, through my therapy session. No comment about the missing tube. At last Charles finishes, and Mother, Yvonne, and I head back to my room. The three of us are sitting here, Yvonne and I looking at one another and smiling knowingly. Still Mother doesn't notice that it is gone!

Finally Yvonne hints: "Sue's nose certainly looks better today, doesn't it?"

"Sue! Your nose. The tube is gone! Sue, that dreadful tube is finally gone!"

Poor Mother is ecstatic, yet she is very upset at not having noticed. But watching me in therapy every afternoon, holding back the tears, is so disturbing for her that she has difficulty focusing on anything else. Now she smiles. We all do.

What a surprise when our associate pastor, Paul, walks into my room. This is the first time he's been here since Christmas Day. I've wondered about Paul, wondered why he has never come back. I even asked about him on occasion during San's weekly visits. Hospital calls aren't Paul's responsibility, of course, but we've known him well, and he *did* come that one time.

"I'll be leaving St. Philip soon, and I couldn't go without seeing you to say good-bye." Paul was getting his first senior pastorate.

"I feel terrible, Sue, that I haven't been back all these months." His voice is slow and thoughtful. "This is the first time that I could make myself come again. I want to explain that to you."

"That's not necessary, Paul. I understand."

"No, you don't, Sue," he says. "You see, when I was a youngster, my mother had a very serious illness. For some reason, when I saw you on Christmas Day, you reminded me of her." His expression is sad. "I'm embarrassed to tell you this, but I couldn't face that again. In my years of ministry, I've handled everything I had to handle, but I couldn't deal with this. Can you ever forgive me?"

"Of course, Paul. I do understand, and there's nothing to forgive."

He relaxes now, and our conversation flows freely. For the first time I am getting to know this fine young man. I admire him for the courage it took to come and tell me what he did.

To Charles, knowing me for a long time as only a helpless object with expressive eyes, my reemerging personality is a shock.

Though I have never mentioned any aversion to "colorful" language, Charles immediately senses a propriety. One of the other patients in PT is a woman with a rather vivid vocabulary. She is angry, and perhaps frightened, about her condition and her seemingly slow progress toward recovery. I can certainly empathize with that impatience. Charles has her doing some stretching exercises that she finds difficult, and she expresses her exasperation strongly—to put it mildly.

"Be quiet," Charles scolds her, "there's a lady in the room."

I can't hear her response, only her grumble. But Charles is firm. "I hurt Sue much more than I do you, and she doesn't talk to me like that."

I feel bad for her. He does not know how much pain she is experiencing, and she surely does not mean to bother anyone else. After she leaves, Charles returns to work on me again and he apologizes for her. This amuses me, since Charles's vocabulary has a few choice words that slip from his mouth on some occasions.

In addition to my spoken words, Charles is discovering that body language says a great deal. Sometimes even my meager movements evoke surprise from him. I am sitting waiting for our next workout. One hand crosses over my lap and rests atop the other at my right side.

Charles studies me, tipping his head and raising an eyebrow. "Oh, my. Look at you! A real lady."

I feel myself blush. It has been so long since anyone observed me as a lady.

In my room after therapy, Yvonne opens a large sack she's been carrying. From it she pulls a *Vogue* magazine.

"Is this something you maybe used to read, Sue?"

I can feel my face lighting up.

"I saw this on the newsstand today and I thought you might enjoy looking at it."

She pulls the eating tray over in front of me and places my glasses on my face. While I spend my miserable time sitting in the wheelchair, we share *Vogue*. For ages I haven't seen any magazines, let alone *Vogue*. What fun to look at clothing and all the new styles!

"Well, what have we here?" Charles has come in to put me

back in bed, and his eyebrows shoot up in surprise. This is the first time he's seen me wearing glasses. Plus he cannot fathom why anyone would read *Vogue* magazine. He considers the whole scene quite hilarious.

It is the little things that keep us laughing and help make life bearable. The nurses and I frequently laugh about Dr. Lohmann and The Great Bacon Caper!

Since I love bacon, whenever I have it, I want it left for my mid-morning snack. One morning Dr. Lohmann came in before I had been fed my bacon. My tray was pushed out of the way for his visit. Just as he finished his routine questions and was turning to leave, he spotted my bacon and apparently assumed I was not planning to eat it. So, without comment, he grabbed my bacon and marched out of the room, happily shoving it into his mouth! Since then, the nurses are all pledged to stand guard over my bacon—just in case Dr. Lohmann visits before I have time to eat it.

Of all the therapy I am getting, the work with my hands is still the hardest. Though it is now routine, putting the gloves onto my hands is a miserable chore for the nurses, a job they dread. It is worse than getting mittens on an infant. My hands are still rigid, the fingers fixed and close together. The nurses must powder my fingers and work each one into place in the rough canvas garden gloves. At times, Charles orders them put on at noon, which is even more cruel. That is my precious period of rest and handholding with Bill.

Bill, meanwhile, continues to monitor my progress. Each day I go through my paces for him—two toes, a couple of fingers. Besides raising an elbow to lift my light switch, I can raise one arm at a time off my lap. If Elaine arranges my chairback to a forty-five-degree angle, I can lift my head a couple of inches. But that is possible only from this precise position.

I work every day in my "spare time" to follow through on what Charles has accomplished during therapy. Before going to sleep at night, I try to move everything I can. It takes concentration. I force my attention onto each muscle as I lift both arms and make the fingers touch. When I finish, the hands drop back to the bed, and I am exhausted. But I am doing it; that's what matters.

"June 12: Wedding gift for Mary."

—*from Bill's diary*

Mary has become my regular night nurse during the week. At first I hardly knew her because when she came on at eleven, it was time for me to go to sleep. But I liked her, and whatever I needed done during the night, she did well. Occasionally, however, she works the three-to-eleven shift on a weekend, and this is when we talk.

Mary is getting married. She is happy and in love, but it will be an interracial marriage, and her family has all but disowned her. Her brother is not coming to the wedding, and she doesn't know if her parents will be there, either. Mary speaks openly about the difficulties she and Lee are going through over this marriage. I cannot advise her; there are no answers. But I can be a good listener.

Mary is sharing with me the excitement of every bride preparing for her wedding. In fact, she wants me to be there. She plans to send a van to pick me up in the wheelchair and take me to the church! I'm sure it is impossible, but it is all part of the fun of planning.

Mary will have several bridesmaids. She doesn't want them to pay for dresses, so she has decided to make them, a huge undertaking.

"Sue, would you mind if I sew them here during the night while you sleep?" she asks. "I promise I won't let it interfere with your care."

Mind? I'm delighted to share this adventure, especially since I also love to sew. Some of my night nurses read and others do handwork to help them stay awake all night, but this will be fun for me to watch.

Mary brings in the patterns and the material and lays everything on the floor to cut out the dresses. Next comes the pinning and hand sewing—everything not requiring a sewing machine. They are coming along nicely—and they are beautiful.

I am definitely not strong enough to attend Mary's wedding this afternoon, but she and Lee have been on my mind all day. In fact, as Mother and I are discussing the dresses, suddenly the door swings open, and here they are—Mary in her wedding gown and Lee in his tux! I can't believe they have taken the time to do this! They have only a few minutes, but it is dear of them to come to see me.

The girls' summer appears to be busy. Katherine is working at our neighborhood pharmacy again, and Elizabeth also works there part-time.

It is time for the church's family camp weekend at Mo Ranch, and Bill has arranged for the girls to go with a friend of ours. I am sorry to miss this. We've gone there for years, and it is always a lovely long weekend shared with our church friends and their families.

June is here, and with it Katherine's birthday. Another special family day. I struggle with the tears and fight to escape the sadness. It cannot be nineteen years, but it is hard to remember a time before Katherine, a time when I wasn't a mother.

When Katherine was due, so was Father's Day. I was sure our baby would be here on time, so I decided Bill must have a gift for his first Father's Day. Pocket handkerchiefs were all I could afford, but I knew he'd be pleased.

I had a noon appointment with the doctor on Friday, June 15. This would be it, I knew. He'd informed me that if I was ready, I would go straight to the hospital. So I had my hair done that Friday morning, and my bag was packed and in the car. When I walked into the doctor's office, I was ready to have my first baby. Even Katherine, it seemed, was ready: I was starting to dilate. So off we went to the hospital—where we began the wait.

The doctor had a ranch where he liked to spend weekends,

most especially the Father's Day weekend. But Katherine was stalling, threatening to delay his departure. So, as was common practice at that time, he induced labor. She was born that Friday evening, and I had the wonderful, healthy baby I'd planned for—in time for Bill's Father's Day.

Tonight, I want to celebrate. After all, I brought her into the world. I have reason to celebrate. But I need only look around me to realize how foolish an idea that is. Next year, I announce to myself, we'll celebrate together—Katherine's birthday and all these other special occasions. Then I will be home and life will be normal again—with all of this just a memory.

But for now, Father's Day is just around the corner, and I must have Mother get something for me to give Bill—some Dutch cheese, perhaps. He will like that.

"June 22: Sue's birthday! Melancholy. Teary."
—from Bill's diary

It is almost too much all at once—Katherine's birthday, Father's Day, and now my birthday, my forty-fifth. I am too depressed to feel anything about my age.

Charles arrives as usual with his early-morning cup of coffee. "Happy birthday, Sue." He takes a sip from his cup, still smiling. "You know, of course, that we still do business as usual today."

I knew he'd handle it just this way—pretending to be unconcerned. I also know I need the therapy and will get the full treatment, every painful move and turn. Not fair!

Still, the second-floor staff members all come in with their greetings, which is nice. A number of people ask my age, and all of them express surprise. "You can't be that old," they say. Some want to know the ages of my children, still not believing I can be forty-five. I am pale and gaunt, and I don't look forty-five? It is nice to hear and is repeated often enough that I have to believe it. But why?

"You don't have any lines," one nurse observes. That can't be. I had crow's feet and all the typical lines of middle age when I was home. In fact, I thought I had more than usual because of the brutally dry winter air in Holland, where I picked up some premature lines that never went away.

A mirror tells me that they are telling the truth. All the lines are gone. All these months on my back have given me a face-lift. Is there actually some fringe benefit of this terrible disease?

During my morning workout, I try to escape the anguish by remembering my birthday celebration on the Rhine River—following our first trip to The Hague—when I had about five hundred rollicking Germans singing "Happy Birthday" to me amid the spectacular scenery of the Rhine Valley. Now, here I am at the opposite end of the spectrum.

Even after lunch, Charles is going through all the usual paces. Several people stop by to extend greetings—which is certainly more recognition than I'm getting from Charles this afternoon. I feel a great burst of self-pity.

Finally he says to Ginnie, "Being the day it is, do you suppose we should let up on her a little bit?"

"Oh, I think so," Ginnie answers. Elaine has disappeared, so Charles and Ginnie wheel me back upstairs. There in my room is a huge decorated cake from Elaine, and all the station nurses are waiting for me. Yvonne has come in early to join us, and they all sing "Happy Birthday." Through my tears I smile with love at their thoughtfulness.

A beautiful nosegay arrives, sent by an acquaintance who has suffered a great deal of illness and wants me to have something special on my birthday. Cards, flowers, and plants pour in—and gifts. Ginnie hands me a folding stained-glass plaque in lovely shades of my favorite greens. It bears the verse, TO EVERYTHING THERE IS A SEASON, AND A TIME TO EVERY PURPOSE UNDER HEAVEN. Her gift touches me; again tears overpower thank-yous. What a lovely reminder that even my life here has a season and a purpose.

Charles helps me blow out the candles on my cake—I don't have the lung power to do it alone, but I most certainly want my birthday wish to come true this year: to go home soon! People stop by my room from physical therapy and respiratory therapy, and even from ICU. The stream continues through Bill's visit and late into the night.

Finally everything is quiet, and I am ready to sleep. I'd dreaded this day, but all these people have transformed it into a beautiful occasion. Unconsciously, I've begun thinking of the staff here as family; today they let me know I am part of their family, also. This was a terrible place to celebrate a birthday, but they went all out to make it a festive day for me. If I have to be sick, this is the best place to be.

19

My fingers are not bending, even though I am using the gloves regularly.

We have just finished afternoon therapy when a man appears, announcing himself as a "brace man." He exhibits an enormous pair of ugly metal hand braces. Abruptly, he puts one on each of my hands, forcing my fingers to bend into the ghastly contraptions. As metal digs into the unyielding fingers, I gasp. These monsters are so large on my long, narrow hands that they resemble something more appropriate for the hands of a boxer. The brace man doesn't say who ordered these treacherous demons, and I am too flabbergasted to think of asking.

"Keep these on all night," are his parting words.

Within the hour I am nearly in tears, but Yvonne charts his command reluctantly as an order. Fortunately, she has to remove the gloves several times during our evening routine, but each time she replaces them, it is more difficult.

The pain is excruciating by eleven o'clock, when Patti comes on duty. Painkillers do no good.

"May I read to you, Sue?" Patti glances toward the Bible she has picked up. "Perhaps we can find solace here." I nod.

Scripture has always comforted me, but not tonight. I try to listen and concentrate on the words, but they cannot penetrate my mind.

Once an hour Patti releases the torturous metal gloves for a few minutes, because she can't bear to watch my suffering. Her eyes fill with tears each time she has to retighten them. "I wish I could leave them off, Sue," she says, "but I can't. I could get fired for not following orders." Sadness dims her attempted smiles. My agony has become hers.

I would never ask her to remove them. If this is what it takes to get me well, I will endure it somehow. But I cry all night, and Patti continues her Scripture readings.

"Those don't fit you, Sue," Bill says when he comes in at seven. "Look, they don't fit your hands." I can scarcely see anything by now—my eyes are tired and swollen from tears.

The braces, indeed, are not sized for my hands, and the PT staff agrees. And, after I get the proper size, they should be worn only for short periods in the beginning. Why did that man demand that these be left on all night? To think that all the agony was unnecessary. Who ordered them and gave him his instructions? No one seems to know. Tonight, they say, I can let my hands rest. Are my tears from anger or relief? At least tonight I can sleep.

As we return from therapy, Dr. Gehrken comes down the hall. He is an orthopedist who treated the girls and me several times over the years. A welcome, familiar face! I'd wondered why he or some other orthopedic specialist wasn't in on my case—to avoid mistakes such as yesterday's. If nobody else will ask Dr. Gehrken to work with me, I will have to do it myself.

"Dr. Gehrken, can you do something with my hands?" His face saddens and his touch is compassionate as he examines my red, raw hands and the "knuckle-busters," as everyone calls them. His questions are few.

"You are quite right, Sue. They don't fit your hands. And you do need something to get those fingers bent." He is kind and gentle, just as he's always been with us. "Don't you worry. I'll make you something that will fit and be more comfortable."

Though I am relieved, I still wonder—why did I have to take the initiative and hire my own orthopedist?

"June 28: Ask Sue about things I should have pushed for."
—from Bill's diary

The hole in my neck left by the tracheostomy tube is only a pinhole from the outside, but Dr. Lohmann says scar tissue has built up inside and it isn't closing naturally. It will have to be repaired surgically.

"Can they do it in my room, like the draining of my lungs?"

"No, you'll have to go to surgery. It will be a local," he says, "a very routine procedure. Nothing to worry about."

So much has happened to me already that I am apprehensive. "Can you go with me to surgery, Elaine, please?" If Elaine is with me, I know I'll be all right.

Usually private-duty nurses are not allowed in surgery. But Elaine is resourceful. "I have a couple of friends who work in surgery. I'll see what I can do."

Elaine arrives for work dressed in her surgical greens. This is the first time I have seen her without her white uniform. With her red hair, she looks pretty in green. I feel at ease as she rolls me off to the operating room.

With the blockage repaired, I am at last able to cough up the accumulated phlegm. It hurts, but it is a relief. Now it will be just a couple of days and I can go in the Hubbard tank!

Bill has looked at the tank and neither he nor I can figure out how I will be put into it. All we can think is that Elaine probably will have to go in the water with me. If both of us are in wet swimsuits, it is certainly going to be difficult to dry and dress me. But my husband has an idea.

Elaine and I stare in disbelief as Bill proudly pulls rubber waders out of a sack and hands them to her. "These are for you!" he announces to Elaine. "I got the smallest size they had." He has been to a surplus store and found the boots that hunters and fishermen use to wade into deep water. Elaine and I roll with laughter. The boots would probably be chest-high on a short man, but tiny Elaine could get lost in them.

Charles makes it clear: "No one but Sue goes in the tank." Evidently he has a plan, but I still wonder.

Now we have another problem: My old swimsuit is now way too large for me. I quickly send Elizabeth shopping for a two-piece suit that will cover me fully—a tall order, but she finds one, and I am ready for the tank!

I am excited thinking about that warm bath, but, as with any unknown, I am also apprehensive. I can't wait to feel the water, but I worry whether the catheter plug will work as Elaine explained it to me. I trust her, but I have so many questions. How much will my bladder hold? For how long? We don't know how long Charles will keep me in the water. Does she realize this will be right after breakfast? Do I dare drink juice and coffee? Do we have everything we need to take along with us?

Charles has decided I should come to PT in my swimsuit. Can Elaine get the suit on and off my stiff body? After my time in the tank, Elaine will dry me off and dress me in a screened-off area next to the tank. Will they have a bed for me to lie on while she works with me? None of this should be my concern—I can't do anything but be there—but I feel the need to fuss over every detail. This is a big unknown.

"July 6: Apprehension. But tank OK."

—*from Bill's diary*

It's like preparing to go to the beach. Elaine has pulled the two-piece suit on me, both parts up from the bottom. I can't raise my arms enough for anything to go over my head. She checks to make sure I am completely covered by the suit. I am modest about such things, and thankful the new suit offers the protection I hoped for. Just being in the suit is a thrill—at last something other than a hospital gown! It's pretty—black with pink, green, and yellow dots. I feel dressed up!

Elaine has packed up towels, a shower cap, hospital gown, brush, and the Foley—to hook me up again as soon as I am out of the tank.

Charles comes to my room pushing a litter cart like those used to take patients to surgery.

"You can't take me down on that, Charles." That looks to me like a big step backward.

"Sorry, Sue, that's what we have to do." On top of the cart is a stretcher, which will be used to transfer me into the tank. I don't like the sound of this at all.

"We'll leave now, Elaine," he says to her as soon as I am positioned on the cart, "and you just come down whenever you're ready."

I shoot a glance at Elaine. Oh, no, you don't, Charles. I want her along with me now. This is as new an experience for Charles as it is for us. I need the security of Elaine. She packs my belongings onto the wheelchair and follows us to the elevator.

Charles shows off the now-steaming Hubbard tank and then straps me to the stretcher. Carefully he and Richard lift the stretcher off the cart and lower me into the water.

Only a long, throaty sigh escapes my lips as I experience the ecstasy of the warm water covering my body. After all this time, I must be in heaven.

Just as on the day I first spoke, it seems that the whole hospital staff is swarming in to look at Sue in the tank—Sue beaming gleefully.

"Hey, look who's swimming!"

"How's the water, Sue?"

"Wonderful!" is all I can respond.

A doctor saunters in. "Why, there's Esther Williams!" Everyone laughs. For the moment, that's who I feel like.

For this first immersion, Charles says all I have to do is lie here and enjoy it, and I do. I don't ever want to be taken out. The jets propel water at me from every direction. The shower cap flies off, but I don't care if my head gets wet. Every drop of water feels magnificent.

During the first days in the tank, we do only the routine movements that Charles and I have worked with on the table—crossing my arms and then my legs and stomach-muscle exercises. These go much better in the tank. Gradually we begin more aggressive work. The first time Charles flops me over on my side, I am startled. My head is still out of the water, and he is right here, but this huge tank of water looks different, almost foreboding from this position. I feel vulnerable, knowing I can't move anything well enough to swim.

"July 15: Frustrated and depressed again."
—from Bill's diary

As with every high, the low always follows. Again I feel myself sinking. This illness has gone on too long, and improvement is less noticeable. Months back, I clung to one thought: Get out of intensive care and get in the tank and everything will turn around.

But it isn't working that way. Little frustrations grow into major irritations. I still can do nothing for myself. Nurses whom I have cherished as friends become irritating. Having everything done for me is wearing thin. Every bodily function is tended to when it suits someone else. I eat when the tray comes, and I eat what the hospital gives me, spooned into my mouth by someone else's hand. Time on the commode is assigned. Face washing, tooth brushing—everything is still done for me. I want desperately to be able to take care of myself.

And I have been away from home too long. Bill and the girls are getting tense with each other. I have always been the one who kept things going. Now Bill is having to monitor their schedules. Tempers flare. He never had to deal with all that before. I always knew ahead what they had planned and asked, "Now, what are you going to need for this?" I foresaw problems so that we wouldn't have frantic, down-to-the-last-minute episodes. I need to get back home to assume my role again as a full-time wife and mother. The three months that once sounded like a life sentence have come and gone. After 7½ months, I am still helpless. The hundreds of disappointments are overwhelming me. In ICU I fought fear and anger. Now I battle depression—and the constant, demoralizing pain of the gloves, the wheelchair, therapy.

Every morning I wake up dreading therapy—more pain, more fear, and always more tears. I have never once doubted that Charles cares deeply about me—after all, he never misses that early-morning visit with his cup of coffee. But as he leaves, I know I'll soon be with him in therapy, and he'll be hurting me again. I can't get well without him, but still there is dread.

Now Charles is prodding me to do more on my own. I am using every free minute to work myself—trying, trying, and trying again to push for more movement. Still he demands and reminds. Why won't my friend believe I am doing all I can?

The summer is dragging on—long and sad.

"July 23: Anniversary. 21 years."

—from Bill's diary

I seek out quiet places in my thoughts to shelter me from the reality of my life and the desperate sadness of being here on this special day. So many years ago, our wedding day, yet in my memories it remains real, warm and lovely. I can still picture Bill's parents when they arrived in Richmond the day before our wedding.

I'd never before been around anyone who spoke with a New Jersey accent. Bill didn't have one. I had met the Baiers only by telephone; now I was finally meeting them in person. They were as kind and loving as I knew they would be. But listening to them talk was a totally new sound experience. It didn't occur to me at the time that I might sound just as strange to them.

Our wedding was a seven o'clock candlelight ceremony. The moment came. I clung to Daddy's arm and felt myself tensing when I looked down the aisle. Then I saw Bill, smiling at me. It was a beautiful, big smile! I didn't see anyone else in the church.

The service was followed by a reception at the country club, around the pool. It was a hot, sticky July evening, and the mosquitoes were fearsome. This was the first time I'd met Bill's brother-in-law, John. Just prior to our forming the receiving line, he saw all the mosquitoes stuck in my veil. Off he went to find a can of bug spray. We've laughed with him ever since about the dousing he gave me—such an aroma for a new bride!

Bill came to the hospital this morning early. His smile still obscures everyone in a room. All I could do was cry. What kind of anniversary was this? Was I ever going to get out of this hospital? The day is heartbreaking.

Katherine, Elizabeth, and Lissy have come up with a surprise for us, a gala dinner party for two. They arrive bearing a cake, flowers, candles, and fresh, boiled shrimp! After much fluttering about, setting up our dinner table, the girls and Yvonne leave. Bill and I are alone in the candlelight for our anniversary dinner. Their excitement lingers, setting a happy mood. Dinner is leisurely as Bill feeds me each tiny bite. Tonight it does not matter that the chewing is so slow—all the more time to savor the taste of the shrimp.

It is a night for remembering, and a night for laughter. Simultaneously we look at each other and say, "Remember twelve-and-a-half!" More laughter.

The Dutch make a big occasion of the twelve-and-a-half anniversary, just in case the couple doesn't make it to the twenty-fifth. They even have special greeting cards for it. Since we arrived in Holland just in time for our twelfth anniversary, we soon learned we had just six months to wait for this unusual occasion. We did celebrate the anniversary, even though we had every intention of making it to twenty-five!

It is quiet now. Bittersweet nostalgia sweeps over us. How very thankful I am for this wonderful man and for our family. How lucky we have each other, yet how sad that we have to be here for this day. Bill stays a long time, but the inevitable comes. As he walks out the door, the tears again flow.

Britain's royal wedding is upon us, and Patti and I are looking forward to seeing it on television. During afternoon therapy, I hint to Charles, "Are you going to stay up tonight and watch the wedding?" I want him to tell me I can stay awake for it.

"No, I'm not interested in anything like that." He may well

have guessed why I am asking, and he certainly knows that I'll be useless in therapy without a night's sleep. Permission is denied by omission.

At eleven, Patti comes on duty. She has been to a pastry shop and bought an assortment of little tarts. The box is tied daintily with a silk ribbon. She has china cups and saucers and special tea bags. She is excited; we are going to have a tea party and watch the wedding of Charles and Diana.

I hesitate to tell her. "Charles doesn't want me to stay up and watch. I'll just have to see it tomorrow."

Patti is crestfallen. "Oh, Sue, come on. This is the only time they're ever going to get married. You've got to see it tonight, live."

But therapy is too difficult now. Charles would know immediately if I had no sleep, and it would be very rough. Patti will have to do it without me.

I have her hook up the pillow speaker so she can listen by herself, but I know how disappointing it is for her to have to watch it alone after all her plans.

"You have to turn me during the night, anyway," I remind her, "so, how about doing it when they get to the altar?" She giggles at our little conspiracy, and we watch the wedding vows together. I won't mention this to Charles.

Tension is building with Elaine. Her personal life has become very stressful and is getting the better of her. Here with me, she has begun a crusade to get me doing speech therapy because a friend of hers suggested it. Charles sees no need for it, and no doctor has mentioned it or ordered such therapy. And there certainly isn't time for any more activity in my day. In the midst of all this, I am again becoming restless about my progress.

Elaine has the most difficult shift—intense, so much to do for me, and always rushed. She never wanted to work days, agreeing to it only because of me, and I have always appreciated that. But after all this time, I can see the hours are getting to her— along with problems she has had with her boyfriend, a burglary at her home, plus two car accidents. She has reason to be touchy, but these problems are interfering with her work. Bill has informed her that she must stop pushing for speech therapy. It is evident we are approaching a parting of the ways.

Elaine pauses in our routine. She barely looks at me as she speaks. "Sue, this is my last day. I won't be here tomorrow." I am shocked into silence. Panic seems to choke me. She turns my chair abruptly, and we are in the hall. Everything whirls by. Should I try to dissuade her? Can I? I have seen this coming for weeks. Now I am afraid it has gone too far. I feel numb.

The elevator is crowded; no place for conversation. Anyway, I can think of no words to say. The hallway into PT swallows us. As soon as we arrive in the therapy room, she is gone and I am terrified. Another unknown. Elaine has been the mainstay of my days. Now what? Charles tries to be reassuring. I am disconsolate.

Bill also reassures me that this was inevitable. We will get another nurse. Still I am frightened. Anxiety overpowers me. My fingers are numb and then my legs. What is happening to me? I dare not sleep. Is everything shutting down again? I pray and I cry. What are we going to do? Sleep finally quells my terror.

"July 27: Guillain-Barré syndrome coming back!"
—from Bill's diary

I awake early to fear. The numbness is still here. This can't be happening again!

It is morning. Who will be my nurse? Who will come? Just before seven, the door opens.

"Marjean!"

"Surprise! You're stuck with me."

"I don't understand. What are you doing here?"

"I just took my last final exam at school yesterday, so I'm your new day nurse. It will work out beautifully for me."

For her! This has to be a miracle. Nothing can make me happier. For the moment, I am too excited to remember my numbness.

Word soon comes from Dr. Lohmann. No, it is not a return of the Guillain-Barré. Anxiety has produced the attack of paralysis and all I need to do is relax. With Marjean as my nurse, that will be easy.

The numbness is gone in a few days, as Dr. Lohmann predicted.

I have been forgetting to ask Kathleen about Judith, her cohort of Christmas Day. All of a sudden Judith walks into my room.

"I'm so glad to see you again, Sue," she says. And I am so glad to see that lovely, kind face again! "Look at you, sitting up! When Kathleen and I worked with you that day, we didn't believe you'd ever get up again."

"Where have you been all this time?" I ask.

"I've been out with back surgery, but now I'm OK and I'll be looking after you, I assure you." She is the other head nurse on the second floor, along with Kathleen. Finally I will be able to tell her how much her lullabies meant to me that desperately sad Christmas morning.

Kathleen and Judith continue to stop in often. We are becoming friends. Kathleen is a tease, and she starts prodding me. "Kick me, Sue," she says. "Come on, kick me." I try to get my foot up high enough, but can't quite make it. "I won't believe you're going to walk until you can kick me."

"Don't worry, I'll kick you one of these days."

Everyone knows I love animals. Several nurses have brought in pictures of their pets, and in PT Richard talks often about his dog. But what a surprise when his roommate slips the little puppy through the side door of the therapy department.

I run my stiff, awkward fingers across that little ball of fur. Such a joy. He is a cinnamon-colored terrier, small and precious as he snuggles in my lap. Everything seems calm and peaceful as I look into that beguiling face. All the pain of the therapy evaporates. The puppy licks my red, swollen fingers, seeming to sense the pain as he spreads his warm, soothing ointment. I am pleased I can give something back—a warm, loving embrace. We are both contented.

"August 1: Buy toy for Richard's dog."

—*from Bill's diary*

Summer is waning, and the girls talk of school again. We must have Lissy's luncheon before she heads for college. It will be one last gathering of friends before the older girls leave town. Plans are set for eight girls, and we decide on the menu, place cards, and flowers. Elizabeth paints flowers on a small mason jar and fills it with blue and yellow daisies. Lissy will have the jar as a keepsake.

Katherine has arranged to get a ride back to Vanderbilt, and Bill will ship her stereo and other bulky items by bus. I should be going shopping with her for the clothes she needs, but I am not going anywhere—except to therapy.

My left leg is improving, but the quadricep muscle on the front of my right thigh is not developing, and I need it if I am going to walk. Charles has started using a kind of saddlebag to hold weights that I lift with my feet, in an effort to strengthen the legs. We started with simple leg lifts, then the empty bag, and now I can lift two pounds with my left leg. But in my right leg I have no capability to lift or support anything.

"A normal, healthy person should be able to lift ten pounds each time," Charles informs me. That is a measurable goal, and I am going to do it. Whenever I am lying on the mat or table resting, I work my legs, making myself raise them. I watch when hip patients work on their lifts across the room. If they can't do what I've accomplished that day, Charles looks over at me and smiles. My determination increases. I will get to ten pounds, *in both legs!*

I watch Charles spread a double sheet on the floor of the therapy room. What now? He is always trying something new.

"All right, Sue. Today we're going to roll." I look at him skeptically. I can't even turn over on my side in bed. "You've got to learn how to roll."

Down we go onto the sheet. The floor has only thin carpeting, and it is very hard. Charles pushes me over and over in one direction, and then back in the other. With each turn, every bone in my body seems to grind into that hard floor.

He gives me a push. "Now you do it."

I thrash out with an arm to maintain the momentum. When I manage to flop over, I crumple in exhaustion.

"Go on, Sue, keep going."

Again he pushes and again I drag or throw myself over, only to collapse once more. My lungs cannot support breath for this much exertion.

"Don't stop. Keep going."

"I can't. I have to rest."

"You can rest later." And again he pushes.

If I come to a stop on my stomach, I can't breathe. In terror, I claw wildly and dig into the floor to push myself over.

For several days we continue, and I become covered with scrapes and bruises at every pressure point. Finally he lets up. Now I can practice turning over in my bed—and I will do this, along with all my other exercises, faithfully. I will do anything it takes to get out of this hospital!

My bruising is a repeated problem and a constant frustration to Charles. It isn't that he doesn't believe me; he can see I bruise easily. But he is annoyed with anything that interferes with my doing what is necessary to get me back to normal. Bruises and blisters interrupt the plan. Where can we go from here? What can we substitute?

Alone with Bill, I cry in desperation, "There are so many dumb things I can't do! Things I've always taken for granted, now I can't do them!"

With everything new we try, I become conscious of muscles that are needed and aren't there. When Charles finds a missing muscle, one I need for the next step, he adjusts therapy to work on restoring it—and then another and another. Muscle evaluations are done regularly to analyze the level of return and what remains to be done.

We've only been guessing how much I weigh. Bill says he'll bring in our bathroom scale and weigh me as soon as I can stand alone. My next goal!

I know I am all grins when I walk with Charles holding just one arm—another milestone. As we near the table again, Charles steps in front of me, takes both of my arms, and steadies me. Oh, dear. Now what? Slowly he lets go of one arm, then the other. I am standing alone! I am so wobbly and excited, I will surely knock myself over. The whole world seems to stop; no time, no sound. Just Charles and me standing here facing each other with enormous grins. More tears of joy. So few muscles and no balance, but I am standing—for a full minute. Finally he grabs hold of me, and all the PT staff is here, sending up an enormous cheer! Like a news flash, the word goes out: Sue stood alone! The whole hospital seems to celebrate.

Bill happily brings in the scale and plops it onto the floor in front of the wheelchair. He and Charles get me positioned and steadied. Then they let go. I can't look down; I am afraid to move even my eyes for fear of losing my balance. So I wait for the report.

One hundred pounds! I must have gained back fifteen pounds. We are moving forward.

"August 26: Katherine back to school. Sue sad."
—*from Bill's diary*

September marks more accomplishments to celebrate. My right

leg is making progress. I can now walk with Charles holding my left arm. When lying down, I can lift both knees together.

Charles decides it is time for me to transfer myself from the table to the chair. He stands beside me reassuringly, telling me what to do, one move at a time. I am very uneasy.

"Come on, Sue, you can do it." Always those familiar words. Marjean nods her encouragement.

I think out each move carefully and then do it. Finally, I get myself into the chair!

"See, you did it!" Again the huge grin. This is a biggie, my first move toward independence.

As I congratulate myself, I see that look again in Charles's eyes.

"OK, Sue, back on your feet." He steadies me and swings over to my side, turning back to smile at Yvonne as he speaks.

"Yvonne, you can push the chair upstairs, but Sue and I are going to walk back."

He's got to be kidding. I am still walking only across the room, and even after so short a distance, I am completely winded and damp with perspiration. The idea of walking all the way to my room is incredible.

"We have all afternoon, Sue. No need to hurry."

There are lots of stops, as I stand and try to catch my breath, but I only get a minute to rest. Then it is onward. Charles lets Yvonne push the chair behind us, in case my legs give out completely. How I want to sit down and rest. But he won't allow that. There are railings along the walls, and I try to grab them for added support, but he keeps them out of reach. "That's not necessary. You've got me."

At times I am sure my feet cannot take another step, and Charles practically drags me, but on we go. I am thankful for the elevator. At least there I can stop and lean against the wall.

Finally we make it to my room, and I know then that I will never again get a ride back from therapy. We have done it once, and Charles will not let me backtrack.

Each new effort brings more aches. Muscles are developing. I am aware of each one as it adds to the soreness of its pre-

decessors. Dear Bill has bought me an electric massager. At the
end of our work day, I tell him where it throbs most, and he
massages away the tension. Oh, Bill, if only I could ease your
frantically busy life and massage away *your* tension.

To compensate for my foot-drop, Charles has been taping my
shoes to my legs at a ninety-degree angle. Dr. Gehrken saw me
walking in therapy and has ordered leg braces. Before the braces
can be fitted, however, we have to contact a specialty shoe store
for shoes to attach the braces to. New shoes!

But these are not the graceful, feminine shoes I have always
loved. The salesman shows up with unattractive, clunky oxfords and smiles politely as he asks whether I want black or
brown. I don't want either. Reluctantly I choose brown. They
are horrible and much too wide, but the salesman assures me I
need the extra looseness because of the braces.

Here I am, getting the most expensive shoes I have ever
owned, and they are also the homeliest things in the world. And
they are especially "fetching" with my hospital gown and long,
skinny legs!

Bill tries to cheer me by telling me they look good. He probably is pleased that I am finally getting some sturdy shoes. Bill
always prefers the practical. I found that out soon after we were
married.

At the time of our wedding, I had a proper trousseau, which
Bill assumed would take care of my clothing needs for many
years. We were married in the summer. That fall, Bill had the
opportunity to attend a meeting in New York, and I was to go
along so we could visit his family.

Mother was excited for me. "We must get you some clothes
for the trip!" That sounded logical, so she and I shopped, and I
bought a couple of new fall outfits.

Bill was less than pleased about my shopping spree.

"Why do you have to buy new clothes to go see my family?
That's not necessary." Bill didn't understand the significance of
seasons in a woman's wardrobe. He had always been very
conservative; his clothes were good, but not abundant or varied.
Dealing with women's clothing was a very new experience. He

had quite an education ahead of him. And he was certainly put to the test when he learned that his bride had difficult-to-fit feet—long and narrow, a combination that always seems to translate into expensive! For this reason, Mother had taught me early in life that I'd have to go to shoe sales to afford shoes that fit. But here we are, paying full price for these dreadful clodhoppers I am now modeling—with Bill's smiling approval!

To make matters worse, Mother joins in. "Why, Sue, the color is really very nice."

"September 15: Left leg lifting four-and-a half pounds. Right leg nothing. Shoes seem OK to me. Sue—Too wide."
                                                            —from Bill's diary

In spite of their appearance, the braces and shoes are going to be helpful in walking. However, Charles has had to add four insoles and heel pads, plus layers of padding in the arch, to make the shoes, with braces, snug enough to stay on my feet.

To celebrate the new braces, Charles takes me outside for a walk on the patio. It is a lovely day to be out, although I am nervous trying to navigate in these clumsy boats. At one end of the patio is a little gazebo with two seats in it. Charles decides this is a good place to rest. It means climbing two steps—my first attempt at stairs. As I try to lift each foot, with two pounds of shoes and braces added, I scrape the toes of both shoes.

Charles is delighted that I've managed the steps. The scratches on my shoes are of no consequence to him. But my world has become so small that I am distressed. Imagine! My expensive new shoes have scuffed toes!

Yvonne now has me sitting up on the side of the bed for dinner. It is good exercise for all my torso muscles. As she begins feeding me, the phone rings—a call from her husband. She turns away to speak with him.

I study the fork and wonder whether I can pick up the fork and put something in my mouth. I concentrate and slowly wrap my limp hands around the fork. With all the effort I can muster, I spear a green bean and get it to my mouth. Such a triumphant feeling! I rattle the fork on a dish to get Yvonne's attention so she'll see the bean in my mouth. We laugh and cry with childish enthusiasm. A little thing that means a lot to both of us; another beginning; significant progress toward self-sufficiency.

The time surely is coming when I will eat a whole meal by myself.

20

"September 21: Sue happy, Charles back."

—*from Bill's diary*

Charles went on vacation again, at the administration's insistence. They knew he needed a break from the intensity of my therapy. I, too, needed a vacation, I decided, but no chance! I had hoped JoAnn would allow me a bit of a break from Charles's strenuous workouts. No luck. She kept up the pace every single day.

Charles's smile is particularly welcome this morning. I have missed my friend while he was gone. Along with the familiar cup of coffee, he is carrying a shopping bag; in it, he says, is something for me.

I struggle to open the package by myself, another accomplishment. Inside is a lovely fringed shawl. I am too touched to speak. I can only smile through tears.

Many days I have dreaded seeing this man, knowing he would hurt me. I have shuddered at his frustration when things haven't come back as fast as hoped, or there hasn't been a muscle where we have needed one. But through it all, he has been a dear, caring person, a very good friend. Wrapped in this shawl, I feel surrounded by his loving friendship.

Two hours later, when I arrive in PT, it is business as usual. Or perhaps not so usual.

Today it is a walker. Charles steadies me upright and then places my hands on the sides of a walker. This is scary.

"Come on, Sue, start moving," Charles urges.

I flash him a doubtful look. I am wobbling and my fingers cannot curl around the support bar so I can grasp it. My hands become slick with perspiration. No way can I lift that walker to take a step.

Charles wraps elastic bandages around the smooth bars so I will have some grip. Around my waist he tightens a wide strap, which he holds taut so I can't fall—like a fledgling circus performer learning a new stunt.

"Now you don't have any excuses. Get walking."

I pick up the walker and take one step and then another. In spite of my shakiness, exhilaration forces a third and then a fourth. I really am walking, and I am just a bit closer to doing it alone.

My next assignment is to walk the halls of the second floor over the weekend. With the security of the nurses holding that strap behind me, I slowly inch around the corridor. On orders from Charles, another nurse follows us with the wheelchair, so I can stop and rest when I can go no farther. After making three stops the first day, now I can do the whole circle without sitting. It won't be long, Charles promises, until I graduate to Canadian crutches, those short metal sticks that encircle the lower arms so they can't be dropped. I am eager.

Thanks to Marjean's experience in occupational therapy, she constantly comes up with new ways to make me more self-sufficient. She and the supply department locate a double-handled cup, and I begin drinking unassisted. She pads my toothbrush handle so I can grasp it and make it move in my mouth.

The Foley catheter is finally removed and my kidneys and bladder work perfectly. Each morning it is a toss-up whether Marjean should first take off Dr. Gehrken's painful hand braces or bring me the bedpan.

The PT staff is not beyond bribery. Charles has worked me particularly hard today. All the other patients have gone when JoAnn appears.

"Well, we're ready to order ice cream," she says to Charles. "I guess we'll have to get some for Sue."

She turns to me. "If you promise to stay here and to feed your-self with a spoon, we'll treat you." That sounds like a fine idea.

"What flavor do you want?"

This is the first time I've ordered ice cream in nearly a year, and my mind scrambles for names of flavors. I settle on peanut butter. Of course, Charles keeps working me relentlessly all the while they are gone. When they return, he sets me up and they form a circle, all watching me. This is the first time most of the physical therapists have seen me eat. And I eat every bite, with much cheering support!

This same night I get my first hamburger. It is sloppy, with everything falling out of the bun, but it is a burger! And I lift it to eat the first few bites unassisted.

Firsts are coming faster now. My first shower is heavenly, as is my first barbecue—another mess, but delicious. And my first conversation with Gary Stiller.

As he talks, I begin to get an entirely different picture of this man. We talk about his educational background, about his being required to live in a wheelchair for part of his training.

"Trying it is never quite the same as the real thing," he tells me, "because you know that at the end, you're going to get up and walk out. But it did make me appreciate what could and couldn't be done."

He explains different muscles and how they work. He seems to want me to know that he cares and understands, that he has been aware of what I have been going through. Eventually, he mentions not spelling with me.

"Was I wrong, Sue?"

"I thought so." I feel no animosity as I tell him. The clash of wills has passed. There is nothing more to be said about that. But I am touched by the expression of sadness in his face. He *did* care.

October 10 is Mother's birthday, and I decide to surprise her. With much effort, I pick up a pencil and position it in my hand. With the eraser, I slowly punch the numbers on the phone. I am so excited when I hear her number ringing. It seems as if she's never going to answer. But she does, and I sing "Happy Birth-day." Mother can't even talk. She just cries.

The time has come to give up the tank and concentrate on walking—sad news indeed. That water felt so good, no matter what mashing and twisting Charles did when I was in it. Even my hands felt wonderful when I could put them in front of the jets after having them in the braces all night.

"Sue, there aren't enough hours in the day to do all that needs to be done," Charles explains. "We have to get you walking if you want to get out of here."

I sense progress when I walk around the second floor in the evenings and on weekends. Bill often accompanies me and watches happily as each tentative step grows a little stronger. The exertion is also helping build my lung strength—I can make the journey now without stopping to rest.

"September 28: Home visit for Sue? Who approves? How?"
—from Bill's diary

Marjean first raised the question of a weekend pass in mid-September.

"Dr. Lohmann, don't you think it's about time Sue tried a home visit?" He'd have to think about that. A week later, Bill asked Gary Stiller about the possibility. We were very disappointed with the response.

"He says to forget it," Bill reported. "This hospital doesn't do that anymore." But Marjean continued her encouragement, so Bill has brought the matter back to Dr. Lohmann.

"There's a committee that meets the first Monday of the month," Dr. Lohmann says. "They have to make the decision. I'll present it if you wish."

"Yes," Bill says, with me nodding as vigorously as I can. Marjean adds fuel. "Sue's been here nearly ten months. She needs to try living at home before she moves out permanently."

Dr. Lohmann will check on the pass.

The first week of October comes and goes, and the ball is being tossed back and forth. Dr. Lohmann asks Dr. Gehrken. The orthopedist says he will ask Charles, and Dr. Lohmann promises to speak to Gary. Everyone is passing the buck. But Marjean keeps prodding.

By mid-October, every time Dr. Lohmann comes in to see me, Marjean reminds him. "What about a pass?" Down in therapy, she presses. "Charles, when are we going to get Sue out of here for a home visit?" She lobbies my case everywhere.

"October 15: Going home up to us?"

—from Bill's diary

I am weary of waiting for permissions. I want to get out of the hospital.

Bill is worried. "Sue, we're getting all excited talking about going home," he says, "just like we got all excited about getting you out of intensive care. But remember, I do have to go to the office every day. At this point, I don't know if the insurance will pay for home nursing, or what we can work out." But all Marjean and I are pushing for right now is a weekend home visit.

Charles, on the other hand, has decided I should get out of the hospital altogether.

"You can come in as an outpatient and continue therapy, Sue. You need to get out of here."

Marjean, though, is determined that I need a weekend pass as a trial. As for the future, she casually mentions, "You know, sometimes I do home duty work."

The time is not appropriate to discuss this possibility, but her feeler does not go unnoticed. Wouldn't it be great to have Marjean at home with me until I complete my recovery?

"October 20: Talk to Lohmann/Gehrken/Stiller/Charles, et al. What is Sue's plan?"

—from Bill's diary

"OK. You want to go home." Bill looks tired tonight. His tone is serious. "*How* are you going to get to therapy? *How* are you going to take care of yourself when Elizabeth and I are gone?" Once again Bill confronts me with realities I do not like to face. I will have to find solutions to these problems for myself. But his predictable, realistic questions are a downer.

However, to keep me from getting too depressed, Bill casually drops a little teaser before leaving. "When Katherine called last night, I told her to make hotel reservations for Parents' Weekend next spring. Think you can make it?"

Boy, will I! We had to miss it this year, but I'll definitely be ready next spring!

Word finally comes. I am to have a weekend pass, starting at four-thirty Friday, October 23. I will return on Monday morning. I can't wait!

"October 21: First steps without crutches. Pay bills, make bed-sofa, get firewood, water plants. Buy yellow ribbon."
—*from Bill's diary*

Four-thirty has turned into six o'clock. That is the earliest Bill can get to the hospital to pick me up. I hate losing ninety minutes of my weekend, but Yvonne makes the time pass quickly as she dresses and primps me. I choose a pair of jeans with an elastic waist. At least they won't fall off me. After Yvonne dresses me, she circles me, checking me over. When she sees how baggy the jeans are in the seat, she bursts out laughing. I have only reached 106 pounds, and every time I sit on a hard surface, I know a good portion of my weight loss must have been in my seat! Yvonne can't stop giggling. Fine friend! But I laugh, too, picturing my baggy rear.

Promptly at six, we are down at the main door with all of my paraphernalia for the weekend, and Bill pulls up. I am so excited I can hardly breathe. It is a cool twilight, beautiful. I inhale the fresh evening air and feel free! As Bill and I pull away from the curb, Yvonne waves. Again the tears, and the haunting thought that I have to come back Monday. Tonight, Sue Baier, you must forget that. You're going home!

Evening comes as we ride, and the night lights look different, unreal. The last embers of sunset turn new glass office buildings into rosy monoliths. We are traveling a route that is unfamiliar to me, but it is the trip Bill has made so often. Once we draw close to our neighborhood, I recognize landmarks. But so much has changed—I've been away from the world for almost a year.

Finally we are in familiar territory, passing the service station, our pharmacy, and the grocery store, and then approaching our street.

As we come around the corner, in the last glow of dusk, I see home. That first glimpse is breathtaking. And then I see the big tree in front of the house. Can I believe my eyes? That big tree is wrapped in yellow ribbon!

Tears flood me. What a fantastic sight! Bill slows in front of the house to allow me to feast on the sight before we turn into the driveway. His hand reaches out for mine. "Welcome home, Sue." The most beautiful words I've ever heard.

As the car stops in front of the garage, Elizabeth comes rushing out the door. "Welcome home, Mother. We're so glad to have you back." I can't speak. It's too overwhelming.

I feel strange walking in through the kitchen door. The house smells different, feels different. I've lived here for many years, but now it all seems strange.

"Where's Tiffany?" I can't wait to hold my cat, but she runs from me. Rejection! After all this time, she doesn't remember me.

A welcome-home banner hangs on the mantel in the family room, opposite the kitchen.

I can't believe I'm here!

Bess has brought dinner—standing rib roast, fresh green beans, and baked apple strips. A fantastic meal. As Bill and Elizabeth prepare to serve, I sit at the breakfast table watching them.

My eyes dart around the room, taking in everything. A room that you've known but haven't seen for a year is very different.

Bill and the girls have been doing things their way, rearranging things to suit them or just leaving an item where it happened to rest. My African violets haven't been turned regularly. They are all growing in one direction, toward the window. I see leaves that need to be pulled off. My eyes can't go fast enough for me to take it all in.

It is heavenly to sit again at our table for dinner with Bill and Elizabeth. Afterward, we move to the family room. I am beginning to feel at home.

Finally Bill says, "It's bedtime, Sue." I am too keyed up to be tired.

"So early?"

"It's not early, and tomorrow is another day." He pulls open the Hide-A-Bed in the family room, our bed for tonight. Unfortunately, all our bedrooms are upstairs. This will be a new experience for both of us.

As Bill turns out the light, everything feels suddenly strange. Total darkness. But then I feel Bill next to me, and I know I am home. My heart overflows as his hand cups mine.

"This isn't going to work," Bill announces. I know what he means; neither of us was able to sleep last night. I've become accustomed to a hospital bed, which can be adjusted to elevate my head and my knees slightly. Since I can move very little, these adjustments are important for making me comfortable. I also know Bill wasn't able to sleep on the Hide-A-Bed's uncomfortable mattress. Every time I moved, he woke up.

"Tonight we're going upstairs," he says. I'm not too sure about that. I haven't worked on stairs in therapy. I remember the two steps up to the gazebo when I scuffed my shoes.

When evening comes, Bill repeats, "We have to get you upstairs."

"All right." I've been planning this throughout the day, and I am ready.

Because Charles taught me to raise myself with my arms, they are the strongest parts of my body. "Remember when I sprained my ankle so badly a few years ago? Rather than go up the stairs with my crutches, I went up on my bottom."

Bill's eyes light up. "Why not?"

Going up works beautifully. I hoist myself with my arms, a step at a time. But I haven't figured out how we'll get me on my feet again at the top of the stairs. I don't particularly want to spend the night sitting on the top step.

But Bill brings a chair, and together we pull me up onto it, and then into a standing position—I'm exhausted, but ready to go.

Walking into our bedroom is worth the effort. This room, at once so familiar and so different, is like a mirage. The vision is distorted, changed in ways that can't be pinpointed. Flashes of that last day, as I left for the hospital, jar me. Is this real? Or is it all just a dream?

"It's all right, Sue," Bill says. "We made it."

Yes, finally, I am back in my own room—our room.

The bed is still not the hospital kind, but it is much more comfortable than the Hide-A-Bed. Tonight we sleep.

The return on Monday is rueful. I don't want to go back, yet there is a sense of security once I pass through the hospital's double doors. There will be another weekend pass on Friday. It won't be long, I tell myself. It won't be long until Friday.

Charles checks on the problems of the weekend. "I hope you didn't use the crutches very much."

"I didn't use them at all."

"You must not rely on the crutches."

"Charles, I didn't use them." Bill left them in the closet all weekend. I used the walls, the drainboard, the couch. There was always something close by to steady me.

When I tell Charles about going up the stairs on my seat, he announces a new challenge: climbing stairs.

After therapy, Charles heads me toward the stairwell, rather than the elevator. Then he literally drags me up two flights of concrete stairs. What an ordeal! As we start, I know we'll never get up the first flight, let alone the second. My left hand tries unsuccessfully to grasp the rail, and Charles holds me up on the right side.

"Come on, Sue, another step," he says. "Lift your feet." My

worthless fingers slip on the railing, and I scrape the toes of my shoes with every step.

"Don't keep worrying about your shoes. You have to learn to climb stairs. Come on, lift that foot. Now lift the other one."

By the time we get to the first landing, even Charles is breathing hard, and we are both dripping with perspiration. But he won't give up. He drags me the rest of the way. Finally we open the door and walk out onto the second floor. Everyone stares at us. We are flushed, panting heavily, soaking wet, and exhausted. But Charles is smiling proudly. "Sue walked upstairs today." Walked is hardly the word, but the staff loves it. There is cheering and clapping.

From then on, we do this every afternoon. Charles stands at the foot of the stairs, smiling and rubbing his hands together.

"Are you ready?" he asks.

"Well. . . ."

"Good. Let's get going."

And the same thing always happens as we open the door to the second floor. I stand there red-faced and dripping wet, gasping for breath, and the nurses cheer. These people! How supportive they are.

We also walk more and more every day. Now I have to do one round of the second floor before breakfast. Sometimes during therapy Charles takes me on his rounds. He walks me to the respiratory department, sits me down to rest, then takes me to the other end of the building and plops me down again to rest. He is determined to build my stamina and lung power. It is always exhausting—the physical exertion of trying to make the body move as well as the nervous tension.

Friday comes quickly. This time it feels different. The house is familiar, comfortable—it is home again. Everything goes more smoothly. We've learned from the previous weekend and are starting to develop a routine. For the first time in eleven months, I can use the bathroom in privacy! Someone has recommended using the walker, turned around, with the crossbar at the back of the toilet seat and the hand pieces coming forward on either side for me to grasp. This allows me to raise myself alone.

Monday morning, we are back at the hospital at eight-twenty. I feel tears coming. I don't want to be dumped here! I want to go back home.

The week is going slowly. I am ready to go home permanently. We must develop a plan for my discharge. I can't stand living like this any longer.

Finally, Dr. Lohmann and Dr. Gehrken agree to write letters to the insurance company, indicating that I can be released from the hospital but will require a day nurse, five days a week, to handle my personal care and therapy, and to take me to the hospital regularly for PT. Marjean announces that she will be my home nurse.

"Don't you want to think about this, Marjean? It's going to be a much longer drive."

"No, Sue, it doesn't matter. I'd come to you anywhere."

Now I know we can work things out. Everything is set—well, almost everything. We wait for the insurance company to approve our plan. I am more than ready to go, but Bill continues to caution me.

"Don't count on this, Sue, because it's liable to fall apart," he snaps his fingers, "just like that. If the insurance company doesn't approve this, you stay here. You know I have to go to work."

I glare at him. I don't need this lecture right now. I have to get out.

"*November 5: Go home in one week. Charles all smiles. Sue took evening walk without crutches.*"

—*from Bill's diary*

One more weekend visit. This time I can relax. Everything is set now.

Near home, Bill stops at our pharmacy. "I have to pick up a few things. Want to come in with me?"

Why not? I have to start someplace. This is the drugstore where the girls worked during the summer. The owners had

surprised me by bringing me a plant on Easter morning, when I
first moved into my private room. In fact, it was the very first
plant I received, so it was very special. I want to thank them
personally.

With my little crutches, and a big assist from Bill to get me out
of the car, I hobble into the store. This is familiar turf.

Fortunately, the store is nearly deserted. Mr. Lewis is behind
the prescription counter. As I walk through the door, he looks
startled, then he runs up front and grabs me. All these years, it
has been, "Hello, Mr. Lewis," and "How are you, Mrs. Baier?"
But now he is embracing me with genuine warmth. His wife
comes to see what is causing the excitement, and she, too, hugs
me enthusiastically. It is a wonderful moment, my first public
appearance. I know now that I belong back in the world.

In the pharmacy, how I looked was inconsequential, but Bill is
pushing me to go on to the grocery store with him. Here I feel
self-conscious. This is where everyone in our subdivision shops.
Fortunately, I don't see any of my neighbors tonight. Bill wraps
my hands onto the grocery cart for support, and off we go. At
each aisle, Bill leaves me standing and scurries after whatever we
need. I make it all around the store, but by the time we reach the
checkout counter, I am exhausted. I've always taken this store
for granted—now it is much bigger than I remembered. Getting
around it is an accomplishment I hadn't expected.

During the week, everything has been falling into place for my
release. Marjean will be my nurse and Yvonne is to be her
backup. Dr. Gehrken approved a chart of therapy procedures
for Marjean to put me through each day. She will bring me in to
outpatient PT three days a week for evaluation of our procedures and progress.

Friday the thirteenth is to be my lucky day! Now I am sure it is
going to happen. There will be no backfiring this time. I am
going home for good.

A huge, lovely cake arrives in my room at noon, and word
spreads throughout the whole hospital: Sue is serving.

Staff members swarm in. I feel blessed with so many good

people who care about me—such an enormous family. They are all proud of me, and I am grateful to them.

I watch for someone to come from ICU, but of those who cared for me, no one is left or on duty. The rest all come, however—the second-floor nurses, respiratory people, PT, janitors, and cleaning women. The air-conditioning man stops by, and the staff from the pharmacy. Bill smiles quietly as Patti presents him with another of her little cards. Then he holds it up for me to read: Accept a Miracle!

This is a splendid send-off, a tearful outpouring of love. All afternoon they come. The public relations people snap pictures for the hospital newspaper. Sue Baier is one of their own.

It is strange as we drive down the street toward home. Tonight is a monumental occasion—exciting and very happy. I am remembering the original homecoming with the yellow ribbon four weeks ago. Now that seems only a dream.

This feels normal. A normal homecoming. I am here to stay!

The hostage of Bed Number Ten is home. I am no longer the patient. Now, at last, I can begin rebuilding my life—as Bill's wife, as Katherine's and Elizabeth's mother, as Sue Baier, person. This is a night for joy and thanksgiving.

Praise ye the Lord. O give thanks unto the Lord; for he is good: for his mercy endureth for ever.

EPILOGUE

Five years after leaving Gulfland Hospital, I continue to surprise myself, Bill, and friends with my progress. Today I can use muscles that seemed useless even six weeks ago.

But the struggle back to recovery has been long and tedious. Five years ago, when I arrived home, I was barely walking without crutches in the house. I could not raise myself from anything but the toilet seat and a chair at the breakfast-room table. I could not take care of my personal hygiene or dress myself. Like a small child, I was beginning everything anew— and with the same impatience.

With Marjean's help and encouragement, I faithfully followed a regimen of therapy each day, including regular visits to the hospital for additional workouts and testing. Marjean's background in occupational therapy proved invaluable. She helped me grow more self-sufficient and taught me that I could do anything I set my mind to accomplish.

We all anticipated the holidays with a new enthusiasm that November of 1981. The girls' Christmas party was approaching, right on schedule. While I could only supervise the preparations, I no longer had to send home lists spelled out from a hospital bed. I was writing the lists myself and seeing to their execution—even buying the special dripless candles I wanted for decorations.

En route home from one of our first trips to outpatient therapy, Marjean drove up to the store where I always bought those special candles. She walked around the car and opened the door for me. I was too embarrassed to face this elegant environment, but Marjean was insistent.

"Come on, Sue. I know you'll feel better when you start doing for yourself anything you want to do."

It was an ordeal for Marjean to maneuver me out of the car and pull me upright, but we forged ahead. An attractively dressed saleswoman watched my awkward entrance into the store and graciously offered me a straightbacked chair. As I struggled with my billfold to pay for the candles, she waited patiently and then smiled with genuine warmth.

"My dear, I don't know what you've been through, but it has taken a lot for you to come in today," she said. "I just want you to know how much I admire you for doing so."

What a welcome to the world! I knew I could go anyplace I wanted to go from then on.

Christmas took on new meaning. The music, the decorations, the sounds of laughter pressed haunting memories into the silent crevices of fleeting apparitions. Christmas night of 1981 ended as all such days should, with just Bill and me lingering over the splendidness of the day.

The first Sunday I was home, we sent flowers for the church sanctuary, a token thank-you to the St. Philip family. On New Year's Day an informal church service was offered in the fellowship hall, rather than in the main sanctuary. We felt that this was the right time for me to rejoin the congregation. We slipped quietly into the last row of seats, just as the service began, so most of those gathered did not know I was there. I was joyful to be at worship again with Bill. Tears glistened in his eyes, too. When the service ended, the loving excitement of the entire congregation enveloped us. It was another emotional homecoming.

The continued outpouring from the St. Philip community began to concern us. The food kept coming. One day the doorbell rang, and it was Ruth bringing dinner.

"Really, Ruth, this is getting embarrassing," I told her. Just then Bill came through the hallway carrying a load of laundry.

"Honey, until that man is living a normal life again," she said, "we will continue doing entirely as and when we please."

With Marjean directing my days, there were always compromises and modifications, but few limitations. Lunch out, after workouts with Charles, became a special treat. We carefully chose quiet restaurants with inconspicuous booths. Eating was slow, sometimes messy, and many foods still had to be cut into bite-size pieces for me. But it was a treat to be back in the mainstream.

Soon after we began venturing out, Marjean brought me a gift—a blue pillow to match our car. She carried it everywhere for me. It was months before I had enough of my own "padding" to do without it in public places.

My knuckles were so stiff and swollen that I couldn't wear my rings yet. It was especially disappointing not to be able to wear my wedding ring. So Bill sent me to buy myself a plain gold band to wear until my own rings could slide over the knuckles again. The clerk in the store put the new band on me, but it wasn't official until Bill placed it on my finger that night. Now that I can at last wear my original rings, I also wear that little gold band. It doesn't match my set, but it is priceless to me.

True to his promise, Bill took me to Parents' Weekend at Vanderbilt in early April. I was more than he bargained for, I'm sure, since I was still frail and unsteady. Moving around on unknown turf, I realized for the first time how handicapped I was. Yet the students and other parents accepted me. Some acted as if they didn't notice; others openly cheered me on.

Therapy evolved as I developed more muscles. From increasingly strenuous floor exercises and clay modeling for my hands, we graduated to the swimming pool. Our wonderful neighbors turned their pool over to me. Marjean warned me that she couldn't swim, but she could get me in and out if I could handle myself in the water. I was confident about that.

Being back in the water was all I'd dreamed it would be. Every move was easier and more sure in the water. JoAnn gave us a book of water exercises, and I could feel myself progress in the pool.

By May I felt ready to resume control of my life. The time had come to go it alone, without a nurse. I could maneuver around the house quite well. And, thanks to Marjean's training and constant encouragement, I could handle much of my own routine personal care, plus simple tasks around the house. I could get out of high armchairs alone and stand up by the side of my bed.

I also knew I could drive my car if I had to. Bill had taken me with him when he did some errands one Saturday. He pulled into a large, half-empty parking lot, leaving me in the car. While he shopped, I tried the key in the ignition. It took some doing, but by using both hands, grasping the key between the thumb of one hand and the forefinger of the other, I could turn on the engine. When Bill returned, I was ready for the next step. "I want to try driving."

We practiced there in the parking lot, and, after putting me through a trial run, Bill announced, "I think you're ready to drive." I knew I was, and *that* represented the ultimate independence. Katherine and Elizabeth would be out of school soon, to help me regain confidence behind the wheel. But knowing I was able to do it was a big advancement.

One morning soon after, Marjean called. Her car was not working. I assured her I'd be fine alone. The next morning, Marjean reported that the car was still not repaired. There was a pause, and then it came.

"I think we've both known this time was coming, Sue. To make it easier on both of us, should we just make it today?"

We both did, indeed, know. The time was right.

Walking was still laborious, much harder than driving. In the car, braces gave my right leg the needed stability for accelerating and braking.

I couldn't lean over, so Bill asked me what I would do if I dropped the keys while trying to unlock the car door. I wouldn't be able to pick them up.

"Well, that's going to be my problem, isn't it?" I replied. I just had to move ahead and assume that those things would not happen. I always carried spare keys, but if I dropped those, I might have to ask a bystander to pick them up. Asking for help had to become a way of life.

The first time I went alone to the grocery store, the man who had always bagged my groceries became very protective. He was careful to put just a few items in each bag, realizing that at home I would be on my own getting them out of the car. I had to balance myself and pivot down and around to pick up a sack. My arms were strong enough, but my legs had problems with balance.

It troubled me that Bill was still doing the laundry, so, to surprise him one day, I decided to strip the bed and change the linens. I couldn't bend over, so at each corner, I dropped to the floor and dragged myself up again to go on to the next corner. I removed the sheets from one, rested, then did another, and then started over again with the clean linens. It was a tremendous ordeal. Finally, I stuffed the sheets in the pillowcase and threw them down the stairs. After all that, laundering them was easy. At last Bill was free of laundry detail!

I still experience insecurities with balance when I face a step with no support. In April 1983, I got overzealous and stepped up a curb without anything to hang on to. Down I went, breaking my elbow. That injury set me back and seemed to depress me almost as much as the original illness. I had been going with such a full head of steam that I couldn't accept being incapacitated again. But my friends wouldn't let me wallow in my misery. They were back again, taking me everywhere to get me over that temporary hurdle. That accident, however, did make me cautious about falling.

Dr. Gehrken's hand braces finally did what they were supposed to do. The fingers bent at the knuckles. Now I do exercises to restore the muscles that will allow me to straighten them or move them into any position, and they are improving. Sometimes clerks in a store are uncomfortable when I try to write a check in my awkward way. If it upsets them and they want to take over, I simply say, "Thank you." I understand they mean well. I'd rather allow someone to do what they feel good about doing than to embarrass them. If I handle a situation well, it helps me ultimately.

Even after five years, I cannot get up on my knees from the floor and stand up without support. I can wiggle my toes, but they do not curl under for balance. Nor can I stand on my toes, except in the pool. I still wear simple, plastic braces that fit into different shoes, but Charles has assured me I can throw away my braces as soon as I can lift my toes and turn them under. At home, I now walk without any braces. Another beginning.

I still have problems eating lettuce or foods that crumble. I do not eat soups in public because I cannot clean off my lips with my tongue.

I ride the exercise bicycle a mile every day. The timing depends on where I am in the book I'm reading while I ride! I spend at least twenty minutes on the floor, working my whole body. And we swim for an hour every evening, weather permitting.

There are days when I still feel sorry for myself for things I cannot do, but then I remember where I've come from. I do not consider myself handicapped any more. I enjoy the good aching that accompanies development of each new muscle. I'm conscious of everything new I learn to do and congratulate myself on each new accomplishment. I continue to celebrate the reality that with the help of God, my family, my friends, and the support of an entire church congregation, I am leading a normal life—an extraordinary life!

On February 14, 1984, Sue Baier returned to the intensive care unit of Gulfland Hospital for the first time since her discharge. There were no familiar faces—only nurses who had heard about the woman with Guillain-Barré. It was a strange and eerie walk to Bed Number Ten. No patient occupied the cubicle. Sue moved slowly into the area, touching the bed, a darkened monitor, and a curtain that held no greeting cards, staring momentarily at the clock on the wall and the nurses' station. Flashes of sadness, frustration, terror, reflected in her eyes.

Quietly, Sue gave the cubicle one last look and the bed one more touch, and she walked slowly toward the door.

A patient was rolled into ICU, a very ill patient. Nurses scurried to attend to him. Sue stopped at the door and looked back once more. The new patient was being put in Bed Number Ten. A long look, a deep sigh, and Sue Baier turned again and walked through the door—to sunshine, to freedom.